about the authors

KITTY BROIHIER, M.S., R.D., is the president of NutriComm, a food and nutrition communications consulting corporation serving food companies and public relations firms. Broihier is a coauthor of *The Everything Vitamins, Minerals, and Nutritional Supplements Book* (Adams Media, 2001) and was previously an editor at *Good Housekeeping* magazine. The author of many magazine articles, she currently contributes to a variety of publications including *Shape, Weight Watchers* magazine, *Environmental Nutrition* newsletter, and *Parenting*. A Registered Dietitian, she received her Bachelor of Science degree in Dietetics from Michigan State University and a Master of Science degree in Nutrition Communications from Boston University. Broihier resides in South Portland, Maine, with her husband and two young children.

KIMBERLY MAYONE is the owner of Wow Delicious, a recipe development company. A graduate of Cornell University's Hotel School, she was previously the creative chef for Odwalla/Fresh Samantha Juices. Mayone has been working in the food industry for over fifteen years and recently joined the faculty of the Culinary Arts Department at Southern Maine Community College. This is her first book. Mayone resides in South Portland, Maine, with her husband and two small children.

THE EVERYDAY
low-carb slow cooker
COOKBOOK

THE EVERYDAY low-carb slow cooker COOKBOOK

Over 120 Delicious Low-Carb Recipes
That Cook Themselves

KITTY BROIHIER, M.S., R.D. and KIMBERLY MAYONE

MARLOWE & COMPANY
NEW YORK

The Everyday Low-Carb Slow Cooker Cookbook:
Over 120 Delicious Low-Carb Recipes That Cook Themselves

Copyright © 2004 by Kitty Broihier and Kimberly Mayone

Published by
Marlowe & Company
An Imprint of Avalon Publishing Group Incorporated
245 West 17th Street, 11th Floor
New York, NY 10011

Library of Congress Control Number: 2003116528

ISBN 1-56924-428-6

9 8 7 6 5 4 3 2 1

Designed by Pauline Neuwirth, Neuwirth and Associates, Inc.

Printed in the United States of America
Distributed by Publishers Group West

For my husband, Daniel Scofield, and my parents,
whose unfailing love and support inspire me, challenge me, comfort me.
And in memory of my brother, Jared.

    —K.B.

For Mark Mayone,
the best husband and father on the planet,
with love.

    —K.M.

contents

Foreword	xi
Introduction	xiii
Slow Cooker Types, Sizes, and Features	1
Slow Cooker Care and Safety	4
Slow Cooking Basics	7
Adapting Your Recipes for the Slow Cooker	8
Measurements, Equivalents, and Conversions	9
Stocking Your Low-Carb Pantry	10
Low-Carb Food Products and Ingredients	12
About This Book	15
Recipes	
Breakfast, Brunch, and Eggs Anytime	21
Easy-Prep Entrées	31
Soups, Stews, and Chilies	51
Beef Entrées	73
Poultry Entrées	93
Pork Entrées	115
Seafood Entrées	129
Food for Entertaining	135
Double-Duty Recipes	157
Sauces, Dressings, and Toppings	175
Side Dishes: Salads and Vegetables	187
Desserts	205
Acknowledgments	215
Index	217

foreword

IT SEEMS LIKE everyone we know has some sort of history with a slow cooker. Perhaps yours was a wedding gift, or maybe you bought it yourself when you were going through your "soup phase."

Kim and I have slow cooker histories, too. I received mine as a Christmas gift from my mother during my dietetic internship at the age of twenty-one. At the time I was living in a women's hospital dorm, sharing a tiny kitchen with ten other girls and doing precious little cooking at all, let alone stewing something for six hours in my new slow cooker! To be honest, it wasn't until I was working long hours at a food company many years later that I pulled my slow cooker out of its box and really started to use it. Today, my slow cooker gets regular use and is one of my favorite ways to save myself time and effort, while still serving my family a satisfying meal.

Ironically, just before we started working on this book, Kim had set herself the goal of perfecting slow cooker cooking with her new, high-tech machine (it puts my "ancient" model to shame!). Already elbow-deep in slow cooker experimentation, when this book came along, Kim knew it was fate; we were meant to write it together.

Whether you've used a slow cooker for years, or you can't even remember where yours is stored, we hope this collection of recipes will help rekindle your "relationship" with your slow cooker. And whether your goal is to find more ways to fuel your low-carb lifestyle, or simply to expand your repertoire of delectable slow cooker recipes, we know you'll find the inspiration and assistance you're seeking in this book. Enjoy your low-carb slow cooker feasts!

KITTY BROIHIER AND KIM MAYONE

introduction

▶ A QUICK HISTORY OF SLOW COOKING

WHEN SLOW COOKERS first hit the market everyone wanted one—and used one—for a while. With time, however, slow cookers lost their luster and entered the realm of "appliances received at your wedding that you can't fathom ever actually using." Today, although some people may still consider using a slow cooker as "pseudo-cooking," for most people the benefits of slow cooking outweigh any potential culinary-ego issues.

The "gold standard" of slow cookers is the Crock-Pot, by Rival. According to company literature, the Crock-Pot was developed from something called the "Beanery." However, it was discovered (after much experimentation) that the Beanery was actually better at cooking meat than beans! So, with a few modifications, the commercial Crock-Pot was born in 1971; since then, more than eighty million have been sold. Other appliance makers followed Rival's lead and created their own versions of what's now generically known as the "slow cooker." In other words, Crock-Pots are to slow cookers what Kleenex is to tissues.

Although the styles, colors, sizes, and features may change, the basic premise of the slow cooker hasn't. For over thirty years, home cooks have enjoyed slow cooked meals, and the popularity of this appliance shows no signs of waning. In fact, judging from the growing array of slow cooker cookbooks available today, slow cooking is back on the "in" list, as people realize how easy, efficient, and satisfying a slow cooked meal can be.

▶ WHY SLOW COOK NOW?

LET'S FACE IT, the world moves pretty fast these days, and most of us have less and less time to spend in the kitchen. We want to be able to come home and savor the simple pleasure of a home-cooked meal with our families, but most of us don't have the energy or inclination to start cooking a meal when we finally get home each night. That's where the slow cooker comes in. Without a lot of time, money, or fuss you can have a hearty, healthy meal that's ready when you are.

SLOW COOKING IS TIME EFFICIENT

Today's cooks, who are pressed for kitchen time but still want to serve a hot, delicious meal, are finding that slow cooking fits their hectic lifestyles perfectly. You'll find that most of our low-carb slow cooker recipes require just a small investment of time. Basically, once you've done the prep work and placed the ingredients in the slow cooker, you're done cooking. The slow cooker does all the work, while you go to work, run errands, or spend precious time with your family and friends.

You'll find that most of the recipes in this book don't require lots of ingredients or excessive amounts of preparation. Spending huge amounts of time on the recipes would defeat the point of slow cooking, which is to have an easily put-together meal that requires minimal time and effort on the cook's part. Occasionally there will be additional steps required to finish a dish after it cooks (such as adding a topping or quick sauce), or prior to slow cooking (such as browning beef or onions). This work is typically minimal. With your slow cooker there's no need to hang around the kitchen pot-watching. In fact, checking on the food by lifting the lid and peeking causes the slow cooker to lose heat and hinders the cooking process—don't do it! Instead, get on with your life and let your slow cooker do its job.

For the truly time-challenged, we've included a whole chapter called Easy-Prep Entrées (page 31), in which all the recipes contain five ingredients or less (aside from such staples as salt and pepper)! Plus, to further cut down on time spent in preparation, we've included some tips throughout the book that will help get you out of the kitchen even faster. Finally, slow cooker dishes are extremely forgiving. If you're stuck in traffic on the way home you needn't worry that dinner will be ruined; most recipes can stay in the slow cooker longer than specified (but not more than a half hour to an hour) without any problem. All in all, when you cook in your slow cooker, time really is on your side!

SLOW COOKING IS EASY

Basically, if you can chop vegetables and season meat, you're already halfway done with the preparation steps in most of our recipes. There really are very few cooking methods that are easier than slow cooking. Plus, cleanup is a breeze, because most of the cooking is done in just one pot! Once you've experienced success a few times, we know you'll be hooked on the convenience of slow cooking.

SLOW COOKING MAKES ENTERTAINING SIMPLE

Having a bunch over for brunch? Need to bring something along to the potluck or picnic? Wish you could have company over for dinner after work on a weeknight? Your trusty slow cooker can help in all of these situations. Using the slow cooker for part of the meal not only saves time (you can concentrate on setting the table or cooking additional parts of the meal), it also saves space (there's more room in your oven or on your stove for other dishes). And, because most slow cookers now feature removable crockery inserts, it's super easy to take your dish along to the party, wherever it may be.

Many party favorites, such as meatballs, cocktail franks, and chili, lend themselves to slow cooking. Your slow cooker is also a handy serving bowl for hot beverages in the fall and winter months. Finally, you can't beat a slow cooker for buffet table convenience. Just plug it in, set it on the table, and it'll keep the food warm throughout the party.

SLOW COOKING SUITS THE LOW-CARB LIFESTYLE

There are a few reasons that slow cooking is perfect for people following a low-carb diet. The first is that slow cookers are ideal for cooking the staple foods of a low-carb diet—meat and vegetables. The cooking environment of the slow cooker (moist heat) results in fabulously moist meat dishes that are juicy and full of flavor. Vegetables cooked with meat in a slow cooker become more savory and tender. In fact, if you ask people who slow cook what types of dishes they make in their machines, they'll most likely say meats, with soups coming in second place. These also happen to be two items that folks on low-carb diets can enjoy often.

The second reason that slow cooking appeals to low-carbers is because following a low-carb diet can take more planning than some other eating styles. One can't just open the fridge, grab anything at hand, and concoct dinner out of it. Creating real dishes from low-carb food selections takes time and effort, something that many of us don't have at the end of a busy day. As a result, some people practically *stop* cooking when they're on a low-carb diet, choosing instead to "graze" on allowed foods instead of hassling with revising recipes, or they prepare their food separately from their families' foods. Let's face it, a handful of nuts and a wedge of cheese do not a meal make. Who wouldn't rather have a real meal consisting of an entrée, salad or side dish, and even dessert, as opposed to yet another slice of ham wrapped around a pickle? We thought so. Therefore, in this book you'll find *real* recipes that reawaken your taste buds and rekindle your passion for cooking, while at the same time allowing you to stick with your chosen diet.

Kim likes to say that we've taken the "fear and guesswork out of low-carb cooking," by showing that you *can* eat a wider variety of foods (albeit smaller amounts of some of them) without worrying that they'll blow your whole diet. And, because slow cookers can handle a large amount of food, you can easily plan to have suitable low-carb leftovers—no more rooting through the refrigerator frantically trying to find something appropriate to take to work for lunch!

Our recipes are designed so that even slow cooker novices will have success. What's more, there's nothing magic or extreme about these recipes. They're not all super low-carb, there are no strange foods used, and we've included many low-carb renditions of familiar family favorites. These recipes are perfectly fine for most everyone to eat, so they're great for the low-carb dieter who also needs to feed a family (and doesn't want to cook double meals). It's time to start cooking again, low-carbers, so get out your slow cooker and meet us in the kitchen!

slow cooker types, sizes, and features

IF IT'S BEEN a few years since you've even looked at your slow cooker, or if you've never slow cooked before, there are a few things you ought to know about slow cookers before you begin cooking with one. In general, a slow cooker consists of a glazed stoneware crock with a glass cover. The crock fits into a metal housing that contains the electric heating element. When plugged in, the heating element warms the crock, creates a vacuum inside the covered crock, and thereby slowly cooks the food placed inside the crock. Slow cooking requires a temperature just around boiling (212°F), but most have at least two heat settings (LOW and HIGH) and some have multiple heat settings.

▶ SLOW COOKER TYPES

SOME SLOW COOKER books divide cookers by how they cook—whether the heating element stays hot constantly or cycles on and off to maintain temperature. Most slow cookers we came across were of the continuous heating variety. To us, as long as you know what type of heating method your slow cooker employs (and you follow the manufacturer's general directions for cooking in that particular machine), this characteristic isn't so important. In our opinion, the most important distinction in slow cookers is whether the crock insert is removable or not; here's why.

FIXED-CROCK SLOW COOKER

Slow cookers without removable inserts are far less practical for a number of reasons. First, they are harder to clean: You can't put the whole thing in a sink full of water or the dishwasher (electrical element and cord can't be submerged in water). Second, they are less versatile than removable crock inserts. For example, you can't use the crock on its own as a serving dish.

REMOVABLE-CROCK SLOW COOKER

To us, being able to remove the crock insert is an essential feature. Most newer slow cookers are of this type, and it's easy to see why. A removable crock is much easier to clean (either by hand or in the dishwasher); it can be used on its own as serving dish; some crocks can even be used on the stove-top (a nice feature when you want to brown meat before slow cooking it); and some crocks can be used in the oven or freezer. How's that for a practical, efficient piece of kitchen equipment?

▶ SLOW COOKER SIZES

SLOW COOKERS RANGE in size and capacity from about 2 cups to 6 quarts. The smaller machines are appropriate for dips, sauces, and the like; the largest slow cookers can easily handle a roasting chicken. Medium-sized models ($3\frac{1}{2}$- to 4-quart capacity) are perfect for singles and couples; the large models (5- to 6-quart capacity) are appropriate for feeding families and entertaining. Our favorite slow cooker size is a 5-quart, which holds just about everything we want to cook and is easy to handle and store. This size is also one of the most readily available for purchase. The majority of the recipes in this book were prepared in a 5-quart slow cooker; you won't go wrong if you use this size. However, many of the recipes would also work perfectly in a medium-sized machine, so if you already own a smaller machine, you needn't go out and purchase a larger one just to make the recipes in this book. You may, however, want to purchase a mini slow cooker (we used Rival's "Little Dipper") if you plan on preparing the dips in the Food for Entertaining chapter (page 135). Mini slow cookers have a capacity of about $1\frac{3}{4}$ cups, which is perfect for dips and sauces. They also have only two settings, ON and OFF, so you'll notice that no temperatures are specified for the recipes where we've specified using a mini machine.

▶ OTHER SLOW COOKER FEATURES AND CONSIDERATIONS

FEATURES

Although most slow cookers are fairly simple in design and work just fine for most people, some upscale models offer additional features such as delay settings, digital controls, touch pads instead of knobs, stainless steel "professional style" housings, and even pre-programmed recipes! In general, a basic machine with two heat settings and a removable crock insert is all you really need to produce wonderful slow cooked meals. You may consider purchasing an oval slow cooker rather than the traditional round cooker; it's handier if you'll be cooking lots of roasts or chickens.

COST

Of course, the more features a slow cooker has, the more it costs. A simple 5-quart slow cooker can be found for around $20-$25 (and sometimes for less on sale); a larger model with more features can cost from $35 to $70. Look for slow cookers at department stores, discount stores, housewares stores, and on the Internet. Many times, bargains can be found off-season (summer), too.

COLOR/DECORATION

Before you purchase a new slow cooker, consider where you plan to store it, as this may impact your choice of slow cooker color or decoration. If you have no place to store it and your slow cooker will be a permanent fixture on your kitchen counter, a simple solid-colored or stainless steel slow cooker may be the best choice. If it will be stored in a cupboard or closet, it probably doesn't matter what it looks like, and cost and performance will be the main considerations.

▶ SLOW COOKER MANUFACTURERS

LISTED HERE ARE the major manufacturers of slow cookers available in the United States. You may want to view their products on the manufacturer's Web sites or on discount Web sites before you make a slow cooker purchase.

MANUFACTURER	WEB ADDRESS FOR SLOW COOKER INFORMATION
Farberware	esalton.com
GE (General Electric)	geappliances.com
Hamilton Beach	hamiltonbeach.com
Rival	crockpot.com
Toastmaster	esalton.com
West Bend	westbend.com

slow cooker care and safety

IT'S GREAT TO have a gadget around that will help you prepare fantastic meals with minimal effort, but before you jump right into the recipes, it would be wise to review a few points about how to take care of your slow cooker and how to handle it safely.

▶ TAKING CARE OF YOUR SLOW COOKER

SLOW COOKER CARE is not complicated or difficult. In fact, if you handle your slow cooker carefully, keep it clean, and use it as it was intended, your machine will have a long and productive life. Here are a few tips on caring for your machine.

- If you're like most people, you gave only a cursory glance at the instructions that came with your slow cooker (if you even looked at them at all!). Do NOT throw out the instruction booklet that came with your slow cooker. If you already have (or can't find your booklet) check the manufacturer's Web site for a printable copy of the instruction booklet. This booklet contains information that's specific to your slow cooker, and you may need to refer to it from time to time. It's also a good idea to jot down the model number and purchase date and location on the front cover, in case you ever need service on your slow cooker or have to return it for any reason. You can even staple the receipt to the cover if you want to keep everything in one place. Finally, take time to read the instruction booklet before you start cooking with your slow cooker. Many models have specific "first-time" usage instructions you'll need to follow in order to get the best performance from your machine.

- In general, sudden temperature changes are not safe for slow cooker crocks. For example, you should not place cold or frozen ingredients into a hot slow cooker crock. It may cause the crock to crack. Similarly, do not add boiling-hot food to a very cold crock; cool down the liquid first, or warm the crock by running warm water over it. When removing the slow cooker crock after cooking, do not set it directly in the refrigerator. Instead, transfer leftover slow cooked food to another dish for refrigeration.

- Avoid knocking the slow cooker crock against the counter, faucet, or other hard surfaces. Also, do not use the crock or lid if either is chipped, cracked, or even severely scratched. If you have a defective crock, consult the manufacturer for instructions on how to obtain a replacement crock.
- Allow the slow cooker crock to cool completely before washing it. Washing by hand, using warm, soapy water, is recommended by some manufacturers, but most removable crocks are dishwasher safe. If scrubbing is needed, let the crock soak for a while before cleaning, and use a plastic scouring pad. In many cases, extensive scrubbing can be avoided by spraying the crock with vegetable oil cooking spray or greasing with butter prior to cooking.

▶ SAFETY CONCERNS WHEN USING A SLOW COOKER

SLOW COOKERS ARE safe appliances, and you can be confident about leaving yours at home alone to cook for you while you're gone. However, there are a few points to keep in mind when handling your slow cooker and slow cooked food.

- Slow cookers can get very hot during cooking! When removing the lid from your slow cooker (to add more ingredients, e.g.), use an oven mitt to grasp the handle, as it also can get quite hot. Also, when removing the crock insert from the slow cooker base, use oven mitts on both hands.
- Although using your slow cooker will not heat up your kitchen, the slow cooker base does get hot during cooking. Never touch the base during cooking. Also, it's always a good idea to keep the slow cooker away from the edge of the counter during cooking. That way it won't accidentally get knocked off the counter when it's full of hot food, and no one will be likely to brush against or touch the hot exterior during cooking.
- To transport your full slow cooker safely, secure rubber bands around the handles and lid (use tape if no rubber bands are available). Place the crock inside the base and put the whole thing into a snug-fitting box on the floor of the car. Brace the box with something so it doesn't slide around during driving. Be sure to serve the food within an hour, or plug in the slow cooker once you arrive and keep it on LOW. Some models have a KEEP WARM setting that can also be used until serving time (but not longer than an hour or so). If you'd rather not bring the base of the slow cooker, wrap a towel around the crock, then put it in a snug-fitting box.
- Always remove leftover slow cooked food from the crock as soon as you're finished eating, or within one hour. Cooked food should be transferred to a separate container for refrigeration, and not stored in the slow cooker crock in the refrigerator.
- Recipes should not be assembled in the slow cooker crock and then refrigerated or left on the counter overnight (or even for short periods). This is not a safe way to store most uncooked recipes; moreover, a refrigerated crock is likely to crack when placed in the base and the heat turned on.

- Do not put frozen meat, fish, or poultry directly into your slow cooker. It's not safe for the crock, and it takes too long for the food temperature to rise to a safe level. Thaw frozen meats and fish first.
- Do not undercook foods. Recipes containing raw poultry or beef should cook a minimum of three hours.

slow cooking basics

THERE ARE SOME rules of slow cooking that you should follow, to help ensure a successful dish.

- It is possible to prepare the recipes in this book faster than we've indicated. In most cases we chose to use an eight-hour time frame to make the recipes convenient for people who work out of the home. This does not mean you can't speed it up a bit. In most cases, cooking on the HIGH setting takes half the time that cooking on LOW does. So if a recipe calls for cooking a soup on LOW for eight hours, you can try cooking it on HIGH for four hours. This may not work with every recipe, because ingredients are a factor affecting cooking speed, but in most cases this will work fine.
- Vegetables have a tendency to cook at different rates, according to how dense they are. Therefore, if you have carrots in a recipe, it helps to cut them into small pieces to ensure that they cook through. Only a handful of our recipes contain carrots, so this won't be a factor very often. More likely, you'll have vegetables that need to be placed on top of the meat, or layered in a particular way; this is to make sure that they cook through but are not overcooked.
- It never hurts to spray the slow cooker crock with cooking spray before using it. It makes cleanup easier. Many of our recipes call for greasing the crock with butter. We do this because the butter also adds flavor to the recipe.
- Always trim excess fat from meat and poultry. This helps lower the amount of total fat in the recipe and also makes for a nicer finished product. Nobody likes greasy food! In some cases—our recipes for ribs, for example—we advise you to skim or pour off the fat after the dish has cooked, and before serving, to avoid ingesting large amounts of fat.
- Many slow cooked recipes seem to have an "excess" of sauce. This typically happens because moisture is retained in the slow cooker during cooking, rather than evaporating like it does with stove-top cooking. Not to worry—for most people having too much sauce for a dish is not a problem! If you end up with too much sauce for the food, you can keep the extra to serve on a different food the next day, or just toss it.

adapting your recipes for the slow cooker

IT'S EASIEST TO adapt a slow cooker recipe to one you want to make, but you can even adapt a regular recipe to use with the slow cooker, with a few changes. In general, there are three areas that determine whether an adapted recipe will be successful in a slow cooker: amount of cooking liquid, length of cooking time, and quantities and shapes of ingredients.

Step 1: Find a similar slow cooker recipe. This will help you judge ingredient amounts and cooking time. For example, if you want to make your grandmother's beef stew, consult our beef stew and compare the two recipes.

Step 2: Unless the recipe is for soup, cut the liquid in half. Slow cooking retains liquid, whereas cooking on the stove or in the oven causes liquid to evaporate. For soups, keep the liquid the same as the regular recipe.

Step 3: Brown any ground meat ahead of time (unless the recipe is for meatloaf or meatballs), and consider browning larger chunks of meat as well. Browning the meat cooks out some of the fat and also improves the appearance of meats cooked in the slow cooker. For chicken or turkey, remove the skin first, if possible; it's healthier and looks better.

Step 4: Cut the ingredients into uniform shapes and sizes. If some vegetable pieces are large and some are tiny, they won't cook evenly. Also, dense root vegetables such as carrots and turnips often take longer than meat to cook; put them in the bottom of the slow cooker and layer the remaining ingredients on top. Look at examples in this book for ideas on layering foods in the slow cooker.

Step 5: If the recipe has dairy ingredients in it, be careful! You may need to add them during the last thirty minutes or hour of cooking time so they don't curdle. Again, look to our examples in this book for ideas.

Step 6: Don't rush it! Most recipes in this book take at least six hours to cook, and typically take eight hours. Don't forget why it's called a slow cooker!

MEASUREMENTS, EQUIVALENTS, AND CONVERSIONS

MEASUREMENT EQUIVALENTS

Dash/pinch	=	Less than $\frac{1}{8}$ teaspoon
3 teaspoons	=	1 tablespoon
4 tablespoons	=	$\frac{1}{4}$ cup
16 tablespoons	=	1 cup
2 cups	=	1 pint
2 pints	=	1 quart
4 quarts	=	1 gallon
1 fluid ounce	=	2 tablespoons
8 fluid ounces	=	1 cup
16 ounces	=	1 pound

METRIC CONVERSIONS

Weight

1 ounce	=	28.4 grams
1 pound	=	454 grams
2.2 pounds	=	1 kilogram

Volume/Liquid

1 teaspoon	=	4.7 milliliters
1 tablespoon	=	14.2 milliliters
1 cup	=	227 milliliters
1.06 quarts	=	1000 milliliters = 1 liter

stocking your low-carb pantry

KEEPING THE RIGHT kinds of foods around is a smart way to help yourself stick to your low-carb eating plan. When you don't have enough staple items around, you'll be more tempted to just grab what you can—and in many cases that can mean high-carbohydrate snack foods or carb-heavy take-out/restaurant foods. If you'll be cooking from this book frequently (and we hope you will), feel free to photocopy this list and take it to the grocery store to help you remember those essential items you'll need to prepare these recipes.

▶ PANTRY ITEMS

Canned mushrooms
Canned chicken, beef broth
Canned anchovies or anchovy paste
Canned chopped green chiles
Canned tomato products (sauce, paste, crushed, diced tomatoes, etc.)
Canned or bottled "light" spaghetti sauce
Canned beans (14.5-ounce cans of chickpeas, white beans)
Barley
Quinoa
Vinegars (cider, rice, white, balsamic)
Mayonnaise
Worcestershire sauce
Soy sauce
Thai fish sauce

Splenda Granular sweetener
Nuts (almonds, walnuts, pecans)
Canola oil
Olive oils (extra-virgin and any "mild" type)
Toasted sesame oil
Olives (black and pimento-stuffed)
Roasted red peppers
Kosher salt
Ground black pepper
Bottled minced garlic
Dried minced onions
Tabasco sauce
Dried oregano
Quick-cooking tapioca
Bouillon cubes (chicken, beef, vegetable)

▶ REFRIGERATED ITEMS

Cheeses (shredded cheddar, Monterey Jack, cream cheese, grated Parmesan)
Eggs
Half-and-half
Butter

▶ PRODUCE

Onions
Lemons
Scallions
Fresh mushrooms
Variety of vegetables (cauliflower, broccoli, cabbage); also, frozen vegetables
Salad-in-a-bag
Berries

▶ MEATS

Sale items whenever possible, such as lean ground beef (90% lean), round steak, chicken breast, chicken thighs, pork cutlets and pork chops, turkey cutlets

▶ MISCELLANEOUS

Red wine
White wine
Low-carb shakes/bars/candies
Low-carb tortillas
Low-carb bread/reduced-carb bread

low-carb food products and ingredients

THE LOW-CARB lifestyle is definitely popular, and this is good news for those of us who want to incorporate a wider variety of foods into our diets. Food manufacturers are listening to our needs and desires for more low-carb food options. It seems that every day there are more and more low-carb foods available, both at health food stores and even regular supermarkets! You'll notice that some of the serving suggestions listed in this book include low-carb products such as tortilla chips or bread. We've tried many of these foods and believe that some of our recipes would be enhanced by these foods. It's not necessary to purchase special low-carb foods, but these can make following a low-carb diet easier and more convenient.

We've listed just a few of these food companies and products below; you can find many more manufacturers on the Internet. Many will ship their foods directly to you (order online)! You'll find listings of these manufacturers and their foods when you do a Web search. Using the phrase "low-carb foods" will net you many appropriate sites. Some of these sites, such as www.lowcarbnexus.com, consolidate many low-carb food manufacturers in one place, making ordering extra easy.

COMPANY	PRODUCTS
Arnold Foods Company, Inc. PO Box 535 Totowa, NJ 07511	Lower-Carb breads under various brands
Atkins Nutritionals, Inc. Ronkonkoma, NY 11779 (800) 6-ATKINS www.atkins.com	Various products (mixes, prepared foods)
CarboLITE Foods, Inc. 1325 Newton Avenue Evansville, IN 47715 (812) 485-0002 www.carbolitedirect.com	Various products (shakes, bars, candies)

COMPANY	PRODUCTS
CarbSense 1100 East Marina Way, Suite 223 Hood River, OR 97031 (541) 387-3330 www.carbsense.com	Snacks, entrées, baking mixes, etc.
Inter-Brands, Inc. 3300 NE 164th St., #FF3 Ridgefield, WA 98642 (877) 679-3552 www.branacrisp.com	Bran-a-Crisp wheat bran fiber cracker-bread
JoeBread Foods Company PO Box 42190 Portland, OR 07242-0190 (800) 456-0356 www.joebread.com	Low-carb breads
Keto Foods & Snacks, Inc. 56 Park Road Tinton Falls, NJ 07724 (800) 542-3230 www.ketofoods.com	Various products (pasta, bars, Ketatoes)
La Tortilla Factory 3635 Standish Avenue Santa Rosa, CA 95407 (800) 446-1516 www.latortillafactory.com	Whole-Wheat Low-Carb Tortillas
Lite Harvest Foods PO Box 2292 Lake Grove, OR 97035 (866) 953-9663 www.liteharvest.com	Low-Carb Enchantments cookies
Morgan Confections 5051 Edison Avenue Chino, CA 91710 (909) 613-0030	Allen Wertz Fine Candies line of Simply Sugar Free candies

COMPANY	PRODUCTS
O' So Lo Foods, Inc. 790 Jacksonville Road Warminster, PA 18974 (877) 676-5636 www.osolo.com	Lo-Carb Muffins, as well as bread, pasta, and various snack foods
Russell Stover (800) 477-8683 www.russellstover.com	Low-carb and sugar-free candies
Slim-Fast Foods Company PO Box 3625 West Palm Beach, FL 33402 (877) 375-4632 www.slim-fast.com	Succeed snack bar
Specialty Cheese Co. 455 South River Street Lowell, WI 53557 (800) 367-1711 www.specialcheese.com	Just the Cheese Crunchy Baked Cheese Snacks
Todd's Health & Fitness Products 4003 Pembroke Road Hollywood, FL 33021 www.toddsorganicbread.com	7 Carb Bagel

about this book

WHEN WE BEGAN to write this book, both Kim and I decided early on that this was going to be a book that low-carbers could use through various phases of their diets. In other words, the carbohydrate contents of the recipes would vary; some would have very few carbs, others would be higher. In that way, the book would prove useful to our readers throughout the life of their low-carb dietary regimens. For some of our readers, the low-carb lifestyle will be just that—something you'll do for the rest of your lives. For others, it's a means to an end, and once your weight loss goal has been achieved, you may no longer wish to follow a low-carb eating plan. That's okay. This book is for all of you. In fact, this book can be for people who are not following a low-carb diet, as well.

▶ THE NUTRITIONAL CONTENT OF OUR RECIPES

WE PROVIDE THE "approximate" nutritional content of each recipe, specifying calories, protein, net carbs, fat, cholesterol, and sodium for one serving of the food. The reason that we use the word "approximate" is because, although we've used a well-regarded nutritional analysis program ("Food Processor" by Esha Research), no nutritional analysis can be perfect. Why? There are many reasons, including human error in measurement of ingredients, variances in the trimming of fat from meat, variations between brands of prepared foods, differences in the amount of natural fat in meats, and even significant differences between nutritional analysis program values for the same food! Therefore, although we've done our best to make our nutritional analysis accurate, it still is only an approximation.

To arrive at our nutritional analysis figures, we analyzed the recipes using "generic" ingredient values wherever possible (such as "tomato sauce" instead of a branded tomato sauce). We also used the values for cooked meats (taking into account shrinkage and cooking losses) instead of raw meats, and analyzed drained weights on canned ingredients (such as drained beans and olives). All of these measures help to make our analysis as accurate as possible, so you can feel confident that if you follow the recipe carefully, chances are good that your finished product will be very close in nutrient content to our specified analysis.

You'll notice as you flip through this book that the recipes are not necessarily low in fat or calories. That's because low-carb dieters are not especially concerned with calorie counting or fat gram counting, only with the carbohydrate content of the foods they eat. Nevertheless, in some instances, we've opted to use reduced-fat ingredients such as reduced-fat cheese or "light" sour cream, in order to keep fat and/or calories down to a more moderate level. In these recipes we found that we could "lighten" them up a bit without sacrificing any flavor or texture (or affecting carb counts). In other recipes, we use full-fat ingredients for the best flavor. If you don't want to use these reduced-fat foods, you don't have to; use full-fat alternates instead.

The nutritional information is given for one serving of each dish. The analyses do not include optional ingredients or garnishes, only the basic recipe. If you do add the garnishes and optional ingredients, you can expect that the calorie, fat, sodium, and perhaps carbohydrate will be higher, depending on the ingredient. In many cases, the garnishes do not add carbs to the dish.

Our goal with these recipes was to keep servings at 15 grams net carbs or less. In most cases, we succeeded, but on some we came in too high. We eliminated some of the higher-carb recipes but kept others because they are so delicious. These are special occasion recipes, for sure. Still, it's nice to know that our Crepesagna (page 156) contains far fewer carbs than regular pasta lasagna and can be worked into a low-carb diet with a little planning.

▶ NET CARBS

WE LIKE TO use the term "net carbs," but if you've been following a low-carb diet, you may be more familiar with the terms "impact carbs," "true carbs," or "effective carbs." These are all the same thing: the result of subtracting the grams of fiber and sugar alcohols from the total carbohydrate grams of the recipe. In other words, net carbs are the carbs that count when you're living low-carb. You'll find similar terminology used on the labels of low-carb commercial foods.

▶ PORTION CONTROL

ALTHOUGH IT MAKES sense to keep portion servings in mind, many low-carb dieters throw portion control out the window and just eat until they're full, thinking that as long as there are few carbs, it doesn't matter. This reasoning is correct for some foods, such as salad greens and vegetables, but in general, you should keep portions moderate. If you follow the recommended number of servings on each recipe, your portions will be reasonable and satisfying. Because high-protein foods are so filling, you may notice that you'll get full on portions you initially thought were too small. This is one of the blessings of the low-carb diet—you don't go hungry! In fact, your sense of hunger may decrease significantly. Our recipes list the nutritional content for one serving of the dish. However, if you choose to eat more than one serving of a recipe, you'll need to multiply the nutritional content of that recipe accordingly.

▶ ABOUT OUR NON-SLOW COOKER RECIPES

IT MAY SEEM strange for this book to include recipes that do not require a slow cooker, but sometimes you'll find you have leftover slow cooked food, or that you want to plan for leftovers for the next day's meal. Therefore, we've included a chapter called Double-Duty Recipes (page 157), which contains low-carb recipes that produce enough leftovers to create another (non-slow cooked) low-carb dish. For example, our Corned Beef and Cabbage (page 158) can be turned into Corned Beef and Onion Hash (page 159) for breakfast; our Chicken with 40 Cloves of Garlic (page 160) can reappear the next day as Classic Chicken Salad (page 161). We've also included a chapter called Sauces, Dressings, and Toppings (page 175), which has non-slow cooker recipes that enhance those dishes you do make in your slow cooker. Finally, because every great low-carb slow cooker entrée deserves a side dish, our Side Dishes chapter (page 187) contains a variety of salads and vegetable recipes that don't utilize your slow cooker but nevertheless are a snap to prepare.

▶ ABOUT OUR INGREDIENT CHOICES

THERE ARE A number of ingredients that we use and feel we ought to inform you about why we chose them. We aren't implying that you have to choose these ingredients as well, but we tested the recipes with these ingredients and find them to be successful, provide the best flavor, or be the most convenient.

Broth: We used canned store-brand broth in developing these recipes, because it's convenient. Slow cooking is supposed to be easy, so spending time making homemade broth defeats the purpose. However, if you prefer to substitute homemade broth, that's fine. You may even use broth bases that need to be diluted with water, if you prefer. When buying canned broth, watch out for the double-strength broths (Campbell's brand); they need to be diluted to single strength if you want to use them in our recipes.

Butter: All recipes were developed using salted butter. We used a number of different types of fat/oils to grease the slow cooker crock. If we've specified butter, you should use butter, because the dish requires it for flavor or consistency. We've tried to use cooking spray whenever possible.

Garlic: All recipes were developed using minced garlic from a jar, unless otherwise stated. Sometimes you really need freshly minced garlic for the best flavor, but in many slow cooked recipes, the jarred stuff is just fine.

Meat: Buy it on sale! Most slow cooking recipes use less expensive cuts of meat, because the long cooking process results in a tender product anyway. This is a benefit of the slow cooker, so capitalize on it! Shop the sales using the grocery store flyers, and stock up on (and freeze) chickens, chicken thighs, chicken breasts, "hotel" turkey breasts (no legs or thighs), and various beef cuts when they're cheapest. Also, keep an eye out for marked-down meats. These are cuts that can only be sold by the store as fresh for another day or two, so they'll often have a coupon attached to them. The store wants to get rid of them, so snatch them up and either use them immediately or freeze them for later use. It's okay, really! Ask your store's meat department manager when it marks down the meat, and be sure to shop on those days. For many stores, Sunday or Monday are the key days. To us, a great deal on beef stew meat only makes the stew taste better.

Miscellaneous "gourmet" items: Capers, fresh wild mushrooms, high-quality olives, great pickles, exotic sauces, high-quality cheese, real bacon pieces, and the like all add extra oomph to a low-carb diet and in our opinion are must-haves. We've specified some brands we like throughout the book, but feel free to experiment with various brands, to find the ones you like the best. Stock up when they're on sale, if possible.

Olive oil: Generally, any type if fine; sometimes we've specified extra-virgin olive oil and suggest you use that for its superior flavor.

Onions: Some low-carb proponents deter the use of onions and suggest instead that scallions (or only dried minced onions) be used. We have used all of these in this book. Yes, onions contribute some carbs, but onions also have fiber and other health-giving properties (such as phytochemicals) that, along with their fabulous flavor, made us want to include them. Please do not be wary of the onion; it is an essential base ingredient in so many cuisines, and in our opinion, cannot be eliminated.

Salt: We used kosher salt only because Kim prefers it! If you haven't tried it, consider buying some; it's not expensive and it makes you feel more "gourmet" when you're cooking. Kosher salt contains no iodine but may contain yellow prussiate of soda, an anti-caking agent; regular table salt usually contains iodine and other additives. Although kosher salt and regular salt do not measure the same when using large amounts of salt, our recipes use just small amounts, so you can easily substitute the same amount of regular table salt for the kosher salt in every recipe. Also, we've tried to keep the salt levels reasonable, so that people who prefer their food saltier can add more salt at the table if desired. That way, everybody's happy.

Splenda: We used this sweetener in our recipes. It's made from real sugar and can substitute for sugar in a 1:1 ratio. It's available in bulk form in a box (as opposed to opening all those little packets) and is called Splenda Granular. We hear that a new, larger package size was recently launched, which most likely offers the best value. We like the taste of Splenda, but you may prefer a different type. Be aware that not all sugar substitutes can be used in slow cooker cooking, where dishes are heated for extended times. Check each product's packaging information to be sure it's okay to heat and cook with the sugar substitute.

Vegetable oil: Use what you prefer when we specify this generic. We generally use canola oil, because it has a healthy fatty acid ratio, but any vegetable oil will work fine in the recipes and won't alter the nutritional content. In some cases, we like to use an oil that complements the dish, such as corn oil in Mexican recipes.

Vegetables: We have opted to use frozen vegetables in some recipes, mainly because these are so convenient. We prefer Birdseye or Green Giant brands for their high quality.

Kitchen tools and gadgets: There are a number of tools that we think are indispensable in the kitchen, for slow cooker cooking and more. These include the following:

- Instant-read thermometer for testing the temperature of roast chicken, turkey, or other meats
- Good oven mitts (you'll need them when lifting the lid of the slow cooker—stand back to let steam come out!)
- Plenty of plastic storage containers of various sizes, for leftovers and prepped ingredients
- Sharp kitchen knives of various types/sizes. Have them sharpened professionally once a year
- Ladles: one small, one large
- Whisks: one small, one large
- Liquid and dry measuring cups that are easy to read
- Kitchen tongs: two (you'll be using them a lot!)

breakfast, brunch, and eggs anytime

egg casserole with sweet onion and sausage

▶ **ESTIMATED PREPARATION TIME:** 20 minutes   ▶ **COOK TIME:** 4 hours   ▶ **SERVINGS:** 6

This savory dish is a natural for brunch: It's easy to make and frees up your stove and oven for other recipes. Put it together when you wake up and it will be ready and waiting for your guests a few hours later.

1 medium sweet onion (Vidalia), chopped

1 pound turkey breakfast sausage, meat pushed out of casings

½ teaspoon butter

10 eggs, beaten

1 cup light cream

½ cup grated Parmesan cheese

1½ cups shredded reduced-fat cheddar cheese, divided

¼ teaspoon black pepper

¼ teaspoon Tabasco sauce (about 2 shakes)

1. In a medium nonstick skillet over medium heat, cook sausage pieces about 5 minutes. Add chopped onion to the skillet and cook sausage and onion together, stirring occasionally, another 5 minutes or until sausage pieces are cooked through and onions are soft. Remove from heat, drain off fat, and set aside.

2. While sausage and onion mixture is cooking, grease the slow cooker crock with the butter, leaving excess in the crock.

3. In a large bowl, beat eggs with a whisk, then add remaining ingredients except for 1 cup of the cheddar cheese. Stir in reserved sausage and onions and pour entire mixture into the slow cooker crock. Sprinkle mixture with remaining 1 cup of cheese.

4. Cover slow cooker and cook on LOW for 3½ to 4 hours. (This will yield a moist casserole. If you prefer a drier casserole, cook for 4½ hours on LOW. Do not cook longer or the top will become too brown and eggs will be overcooked.)

approximate nutritional content
▶ Calories: 553, Protein: 39g, Net Carbs: 5g, Fat: 42g, Cholesterol: 488mg, Sodium: 1030mg

▶ **cook's tip**

Vidalia onions are sweet and mild, and won't overpower the eggs in this dish. If you don't have Vidalia onions on hand, you may use regular white or Spanish onions, but only use ⅓ cup of chopped onion pieces. Don't like onions? You can leave them out entirely or substitute ¼ cup dried minced onions in place of the chopped onions, for a nice flavor without the obvious onion pieces.

ham and cheese strata

▶ **ESTIMATED PREPARATION TIME:** 10 minutes ▶ **COOK TIME:** 3 hours ▶ **SERVINGS:** 6

A classic brunch dish, this strata is a snap to prepare, smells heavenly when cooking, and tastes equally divine. It's a substantial dish, so don't hesitate to make it for dinner, too!

1 tablespoon butter

8 slices low-carb white bread, crusts removed and saved, and square centers divided into 16 triangles, staled (cut up and leave out overnight, or toast briefly in a 250°F oven)

6 ounces thinly sliced ham, roughly chopped

8 ounces shredded Monterey Jack cheese, divided

2 tablespoons dried minced onions, divided

6 eggs

3¼ cups half-and-half

½ teaspoon kosher salt

¾ teaspoon black pepper

¼ teaspoon Tabasco sauce (about 2 shakes)

1. Grease the slow cooker crock with the butter (leave excess in the crock). Place 8 of the bread triangles into the bottom of the slow cooker; sprinkle in the trimmed-off crusts so that the bottom of the slow cooker is covered with bread.

2. Add the ham, sprinkling it over the bread to make a thick layer, then add all but ½ cup of the cheese. Sprinkle 1 tablespoon of the onions over the cheese; top with remaining 8 bread triangles and set aside.

3. In a large mixing bowl, combine the eggs, half-and-half, salt, pepper and Tabasco sauce; whisk until blended. Pour the egg mixture over the bread triangles, then sprinkle with remaining onions. Let mixture sit 15 minutes, then sprinkle on reserved ½ cup of cheese.

4. Cover and cook on LOW for 3 hours. Remove the slow cooker lid and let the strata rest for 10 minutes before cutting and serving.

approximate nutritional content
▶ Calories: 552, Protein: 34g, Net Carbs: 13g, Fat: 39g, Cholesterol: 316mg, Sodium: 914mg

---

▶ **cook's tip**

This recipe is easily adjusted to suit your tastes. Try using cooked chicken, smoked turkey, crabmeat, or salad shrimp instead of the ham. You could also include chopped vegetables such as blanched broccoli.

huevos rancheros

▶ **ESTIMATED PREPARATION TIME:** 5 minutes   ▶ **COOK TIME:** 4 hours   ▶ **SERVINGS:** 6

These Mexican-style eggs are as easy to prepare as they are delicious. For a simple dinner, try them with low-carb tortillas, some shredded lettuce, and chopped tomatoes.

1 tablespoon butter

10 eggs, beaten

1 cup light cream

12 ounces shredded Mexican-blend cheese (about 3 cups), divided

1 4-ounce can chopped green chilies, drained

½ teaspoon black pepper

¼ teaspoon chili powder

1 10-ounce can red enchilada sauce

sour cream (optional)

sliced avocado (optional)

1. Grease the slow cooker crock with the butter (leave excess in the crock); set aside.

2. In a large mixing bowl, combine the eggs, black pepper, chili powder, cream, and 2 cups of the cheese. Add chilies and stir together. Pour mixture into slow cooker crock. Cover and cook on LOW for 3 hours 45 minutes. (If cooking time is extended the outer edges might burn.)

3. Remove lid, top with enchilada sauce and remaining cheese; replace lid and cook another 15 minutes, until cheese is melted and enchilada sauce is hot.

4. When serving, be aware that the first serving can be difficult to remove in one piece. Serve with a dollop of sour cream and a couple slices of avocado, if desired.

approximate nutritional content
▶ Calories: 543, Protein: 26g, Net Carbs: 5g, Fat: 47g, Cholesterol: 476mg, Sodium: 591mg

bacon and cheese crustless quiche

▶ **ESTIMATED PREPARATION TIME:** 10 minutes   ▶ **COOK TIME:** 4 hours   ▶ **SERVINGS:** 6

We've given you a few easy ways to alter this basic recipe, but feel free to come up with your own favorite ingredient combinations.

1 tablespoon butter

10 eggs, beaten

1 cup light cream

8 ounces shredded reduced-fat cheddar cheese (about 2 cups)

½ teaspoon black pepper

10 pieces cooked bacon, chopped

1. Grease the slow cooker crock with the butter (leave excess in the crock); set aside.
2. In a large mixing bowl, combine the eggs, cream, cheese, and pepper, then add to the slow cooker. Sprinkle the bacon over the top of the mixture.
3. Cover and cook on LOW for 4 hours. Do not overcook or the quiche will be dry.

approximate nutritional content
▶ Calories: 440, Protein: 24g, Net Carbs: 3.5g, Fat: 36g, Cholesterol: 440mg, Sodium: 631mg

EASY SUBSTITUTIONS

broccoli quiche: Omit bacon and add a 10-ounce package of frozen chopped broccoli (thawed, drained, and gently pressed dry with paper towels) to the egg mixture, then proceed with cooking as specified in the recipe above. The approximate nutritional content of this variation is:
▶ Calories: 379, Protein: 22g, Net Carbs: 4.5g, Fat: 30g, Cholesterol: 427mg, Sodium: 457mg

spinach quiche: Omit bacon and add a 10-ounce package of frozen chopped spinach (thawed, drained, and pressed dry) to the egg mixture, then proceed with cooking as specified in the recipe above. The approximate nutritional content of this variation is:
▶ Calories: 379, Protein: 22g, Net Carbs: 5g, Fat: 30g, Cholesterol: 427mg, Sodium: 487mg

smoked oyster quiche: Add one 3.75-ounce tin of smoked oysters to the egg and cheese mixture, top with bacon, then proceed with cooking as specified in the recipe above. The approximate nutritional content of this variation is:
▶ Calories: 480, Protein: 27g, Net Carbs: 6g, Fat: 38g, Cholesterol: 452mg, Sodium: 701mg

red pepper and mushroom crustless quiche

▶ **ESTIMATED PREPARATION TIME:** 15 minutes   ▶ **COOK TIME:** 4 hours   ▶ **SERVINGS:** 6

This variation of Bacon and Cheese Crustless Quiche (page 25) is great for a weekend evening. Prepare it after lunch and it's ready at dinnertime.

3 tablespoons butter, divided

1 red bell pepper, cut into thin strips, then strips cut into 1-inch lengths

1 10-ounce package mushrooms, sliced

1 tablespoon dried minced onion

¼ teaspoon kosher salt

10 eggs, beaten

1 cup light cream

½ teaspoon black pepper

1 8-ounce package shredded reduced-fat cheddar cheese (or your favorite)

1. Grease the slow cooker crock with 1 tablespoon of the butter (leave excess in the crock); set aside.

2. In a large skillet over medium heat, warm remaining 2 tablespoons butter about 30 seconds. Add peppers, mushrooms, dried onions, and salt; sauté until pepper is soft and mushrooms have lost their water, about 5 minutes. Drain the vegetables, if necessary, then add them to the slow cooker crock.

3. In a medium mixing bowl, whisk together the eggs, cream, pepper, and cheese, then add to the slow cooker crock. Stir to combine all ingredients. Cover and cook on LOW for 4 hours. Do not overcook this dish or the quiche will be dry.

approximate nutritional content
▶ Calories: 430, Protein: 22g, Net Carbs: 6g, Fat: 35g, Cholesterol: 442mg, Sodium: 524mg

▶ **cook's tip**
When sautéing vegetables, always add the suggested salt when cooking the vegetables. The salt pulls the water out of the vegetables and quickens the cooking process.

seafood crustless quiche

▶ **ESTIMATED PREPARATION TIME:** 15 minutes ▶ **COOK TIME:** 4 hours ▶ **SERVINGS:** 6

This variation of Bacon and Cheese Crustless Quiche (page 25) makes a great light dinner when served with a crisp green salad. We used canned crab and shrimp, but you can substitute with any favorite seafood, as long as it's precooked.

1 tablespoon butter

10 eggs, beaten

1 cup light cream

1 8-ounce package shredded reduced-fat cheese (Monterey Jack or your favorite)

½ teaspoon black pepper

1 6-ounce can cooked crab, drained

1 6-ounce can cooked salad shrimp, drained

¼ teaspoon Tabasco sauce (about 2 shakes)

6 scallions, thinly sliced (both white and green parts)

1. Grease the slow cooker crock with the butter (leave excess in the crock); set aside.
2. In a large bowl, mix together the eggs, cream, cheese, and pepper. Stir in the crab, shrimp, Tabasco, and scallions. Pour mixture into slow cooker crock.
3. Cover and cook on LOW for 4 hours. Do not overcook or the quiche will be dry.

approximate nutritional content
▶ Calories: 442, Protein: 33g, Net Carbs: 3.5g, Fat: 32g, Cholesterol: 505mg, Sodium: 605mg

creamy blueberry french toast casserole

▶ **ESTIMATED PREPARATION TIME:** 10 minutes   ▶ **COOK TIME:** 3 hours   ▶ **SERVINGS:** 6

You won't believe this is low-carb! Be sure to use wild blueberries; they taste better in this recipe, and standard blueberries make the dish watery.

1 tablespoon butter

½ tub of soft cream cheese (4 ounces, or about ½ cup)

8 slices stale low-carb white bread, crusts removed (see Cook's Tips)

1½ cups wild blueberries, fresh or frozen (if frozen, do not thaw)

8 eggs, beaten

2 cups light cream

1 cup Splenda Granular sweetener

pinch salt

2 teaspoons vanilla

¾ teaspoon cinnamon

1. Grease the slow cooker crock with the butter (leave excess in the crock); set aside.

2. Spread the cream cheese onto one side of the stale bread slices. Place the bread slices, cream cheese side down, into the slow cooker crock. Sprinkle the blueberries over the bread.

3. In a medium mixing bowl, combine remaining ingredients and blend well. Pour mixture over the bread and blueberries (bread will start to float up). Using clean hands, gently press the bread pieces down into the egg mixture. Let the mixture sit for 10 minutes, then press bread down a second time.

4. Cover and cook on LOW for 3 hours. The casserole will be "poofed" and slightly browned on the edges when it's done.

approximate nutritional content
   ▶ Calories: 532, Protein: 21g, Net Carbs: 12g, Fat: 43g, Cholesterol: 398mg, Sodium: 413mg

---

▶ **cook's tip**

Remove the crusts before letting the bread go stale, if possible. If the bread is not stale and you're ready to proceed with the recipe, lightly toast the bread or heat it in the oven at 250°F until it's slightly dried out.

▶ **serving suggestion**

Serve the casserole with softened, whipped butter and sugar-free maple syrup or Berry Sauce (page 21).

---

smoked salmon breakfast bake

▶ **ESTIMATED PREPARATION TIME:** 15 minutes　▶ **COOK TIME:** 3 hours　▶ **SERVINGS:** 6

This is a sophisticated dish that's perfect for brunch—a nice alternative to smoked salmon and carb-heavy bagels!

1 tablespoon butter

½ tub of soft cream cheese (4 ounces, or about ½ cup)

8 slices stale low-carb white bread, crusts removed (see Cook's Tips)

8 slices smoked salmon, about ¼ pound

8 eggs, beaten

2 cups light cream

pinch salt

¼ teaspoon black pepper

½ cup finely chopped red onion

drained capers (optional)

1. Grease the slow cooker crock with the butter (leave excess in the crock); set aside.

2. Spread the cream cheese onto one side of the stale bread slices, top with sliced salmon. Place the bread slices, salmon-side down, into the slow cooker crock.

3. In a medium mixing bowl, combine the eggs, cream, salt, and pepper; mix well. Pour mixture over the bread (bread will start to float up). Using clean hands, gently press the bread pieces down into the egg mixture. Let the mixture sit for 10 minutes, then press bread down a second time.

4. Cover and cook on LOW for 3 hours. The casserole will be "poofed" and slightly browned on the edges when it's done. When serving, sprinkle a little chopped red onion over each portion, and pass with capers, if desired.

approximate nutritional content
▶ Calories: 536, Protein: 25g, Net Carbs: 8g, Fat: 43g, Cholesterol: 403mg, Sodium: 559mg

▶ **cook's tip**

Remove the crusts before letting the bread go stale, if possible. If the bread is not stale and you're ready to proceed with the recipe, lightly toast the bread or heat it in the oven at 250°F until it's slightly dried out.

eggs italiana

▶ **ESTIMATED PREPARATION TIME:** 10 minutes   ▶ **COOK TIME:** 4 hours   ▶ **SERVINGS:** 6

Break out of the eggs-for-breakfast-only mentality and put this dish together after lunch for a casual weekend supper. You may be surprised at how great eggs are in the evening!

1 tablespoon butter

½ pound thinly sliced provolone cheese, divided

10 eggs, beaten

1 cup half-and-half

½ teaspoon black pepper

½ cup chopped roasted red peppers

¼ pound thinly sliced prosciutto, chopped

½ cup thinly sliced canned artichoke hearts, drained

1. Grease the slow cooker crock with the butter (leave excess in the crock); set aside.
2. Separate three slices of provolone cheese and set aside; chop the remaining cheese and place it in a large mixing bowl. Add the eggs, half-and-half, and pepper; stir to combine.
3. Stir in the red peppers, prosciutto, and artichoke hearts. Pour mixture into the slow cooker crock. Cover and cook on LOW 3 hours and 45 minutes. Top eggs with reserved three slices of provolone, and cook 15 minutes more. Do not overcook or it will be dry and edges may burn.

approximate nutritional content
▶ Calories: 364, Protein: 26g, Net Carbs: 5g, Fat: 26g, Cholesterol: 411mg, Sodium: 768mg

---

▶ **cook's tip**
Use the leftover canned artichoke hearts in a salad. Also, you can add the leftover roasted red peppers to a low-carb sandwich.

easy-prep entrées

chicken with exotic mushrooms

▶ **ESTIMATED PREPARATION TIME:** 5 minutes ▶ **COOK TIME:** 8 hours ▶ **SERVINGS:** 4

Wild mushrooms and chicken make a fantastic pair. Look for wild mushrooms next to the regular button mushrooms at larger grocery stores. If you can't find the mascarpone cheese (a creamy Italian cheese), substitute regular cream cheese.

1 tablespoon butter

¼ cup white wine

2 tablespoons quick-cooking tapioca

1 pound mixed wild mushrooms (such as shitake, baby portobellos, cremini, etc.)

2 pounds skinless, boneless chicken breasts, fat trimmed, sliced horizontally to make thinner pieces

½ teaspoon kosher salt

½ teaspoon black pepper

4 ounces mascarpone cheese

1. Grease the slow cooker crock with the butter (leave excess in the crock). In the slow cooker crock, stir together the wine and tapioca. Top with mushrooms and chicken pieces, and sprinkle with salt and pepper.

2. Cover and cook on LOW for 7 hours. Stir the chicken and mushrooms well to combine, then re–cover and cook 1 hour more. When done cooking, remove 1 cup of the cooking liquid and discard it. Add the mascarpone cheese to the crock and gently stir to combine.

approximate nutritional content
  ▶ Calories: 507, Protein: 66g, Net Carbs: 9g, Fat: 20g, Cholesterol: 208mg, Sodium: 325mg

---

▶ **serving suggestion**

The rich, complex nature of this dish begs for a simple side dish. A mixed green salad or steamed green vegetable works perfectly.

---

chicken cordon bleu roll-ups

▶ **ESTIMATED PREPARATION TIME:** 15 minutes ▶ **COOK TIME:** 4 hours ▶ **SERVINGS:** 6

A convenient version of a classic dish—without the carbs, of course! These roll-ups are also a great finger food (without the optional sauce) when served cold as a snack or lunch the next day.

cooking spray
1 tablespoon white wine
12 thin slices of Swiss cheese (about ¾ pound), divided
6 boneless chicken breast halves, fat trimmed, cut into thirds lengthwise
18 thin slices of good-quality boiled ham (about 1½ pounds)

1. Coat the slow cooker crock with cooking spray. Add the wine to the crock and set aside.
2. Slice the rectangular Swiss cheese slices in half crosswise, making two stacks. Then cut each stack in half again.
3. Assemble the roll-ups: On a cutting board or clean counter, lay one ham slice with one of the short edges closest to you. Lay two pieces of Swiss cheese atop the ham slice, lined up with the bottom edge of the ham slice. Lay one strip of chicken across the cheese. Roll up, starting at bottom edge (chicken may stick out the ends of the ham roll-up). Place roll-up in the slow cooker crock and repeat 17 more times, stacking the roll-ups as you go. (You will have leftover cheese for preparing the optional Creamy Cheese Sauce, or for snacking if you prefer not to make the sauce.)
4. Cover the slow cooker and cook 3½ hours on LOW, checking for doneness by slicing into one of the roll-ups on top to see if the chicken is cooked through. If not, re-cover and cook another ½ hour on LOW and check for doneness again. Serve with Creamy Cheese Sauce (page 177), if desired.

> ▶ **cook's tip**
> If you really miss the standard breading of traditional Chicken Cordon Bleu, top each serving with a small amount of Buttered Low-Carb Bread Crumbs (page 180).

approximate nutritional content (for roll-ups without sauce and bread crumb topping)
▶ Calories: 563, Protein: 80g, Net Carbs: 1g, Fat: 23g, Cholesterol: 230mg, Sodium: 2,382mg

lemon roasted chicken

▶ **ESTIMATED PREPARATION TIME:** 5 minutes   ▶ **COOK TIME:** 6 hours   ▶ **SERVINGS:** 2

This is one of my all-time favorites. It's perfectly moist and very flavorful.—KM

cooking spray

3- to 4-pound young chicken, rinsed, with giblets and neck removed

2 lemons

2 tablespoons olive oil

¼ teaspoon kosher salt

½ teaspoon black pepper

1. Coat the slow cooker crock with cooking spray; set aside.
2. Carefully pierce each lemon six times with a sharp paring knife. Slice the lemons in half.
3. Rub the entire chicken with olive oil and sprinkle the outside with salt and pepper. Place the lemons in the cavity of the bird and place the chicken into the slow cooker crock, breast-side down.
4. Cover and cook on LOW for 6 hours; check doneness with an instant-read thermometer (it should register 170°F). When done, let chicken rest, uncovered, in the crock for 10 minutes before serving. If you like, serve the drippings alongside the chicken for a *very* lemony "gravy."

approximate nutritional content
   ▶ Calories: 676, Protein: 82g, Net Carbs: 4g, Fat: 35g, Cholesterol: 253mg, Sodium: 364mg

---

▶ cook's tip

The servings for this recipe are on the generous side. However, it won't adequately feed more than two adults. It's an excellent "company's coming" recipe, though, so if you want to serve four adults, simply use a bird on the larger side (around 5 pounds), then fill out the menu with vegetables and a salad.

EASY ADD-INS

for lemon rosemary chicken, crush 3 tablespoons dried rosemary between your fingers, then rub 1 tablespoon of it into the chicken cavity and sprinkle the remainder on the skin with the salt and pepper. This alteration does not change the nutritional content.

for lemon basil chicken, roughly chop ½ cup fresh basil. Slide 2 tablespoons of the basil under the skin of the chicken breast, and place the remainder into the chicken cavity. This alteration does not change the nutritional content.

herb roasted chicken

▶ **ESTIMATED PREPARATION TIME:** 5 minutes (plus 12–24 hours marinating time)   ▶ **COOK TIME:** 6 hours   **SERVINGS:** 2

Why pay for a rotisserie chicken at the supermarket when you can have one ready and waiting at home for about half the price? The leftover chicken meat makes a flavorful chicken salad. Check out the Double-Duty Recipes chapter for ideas.

6 cups water
½ cup kosher salt
1 teaspoon black pepper, divided
2 teaspoons rosemary, divided
2 teaspoons thyme, divided
2 teaspoons oregano, divided
3- to 4-pound young chicken, rinsed, with giblets and neck removed
cooking spray
2 tablespoons olive oil

1. In a pitcher, stir together the water, salt, and ½ teaspoon of pepper, 1 teaspoon of rosemary, 1 teaspoon of thyme, and 1 teaspoon of oregano; whisk to combine. Set aside. Place the chicken into a large zip-top bag; pour reserved liquid mixture into the bag and seal. Place the bag into a large bowl and refrigerate for 12 to 24 hours.

2. When ready to cook, coat the slow cooker crock with cooking spray. Drain and discard the marinating liquid, and place the bird into the slow cooker. Rub the bird with the olive oil, then sprinkle with the remaining ½ teaspoon pepper, 1 teaspoon rosemary, 1 teaspoon thyme, and 1 teaspoon oregano. Turn the bird breast-side down in the crock.

3. Cover and cook on LOW for 6 hours; check doneness with an instant-read thermometer (it should register 170°F). When done, let the bird rest in the covered slow cooker for 10 minutes before serving.

approximate nutritional content
▶ Calories: 665, Protein: 82g, Net Carbs: 1g, Fat: 35g, Cholesterol: 253mg, Sodium: 724mg

▶ **cook's tip**
Once the chicken has cooled slightly, use kitchen shears to easily cut the chicken in half through the breastbone.

teriyaki roasted chicken

▶ **ESTIMATED PREPARATION TIME:** 5 minutes (plus 24 hours marinating time)   ▶ **COOK TIME:** 6 hours   ▶ **SERVINGS:** 2

It couldn't get any easier, plus you may have leftovers for a great salad topper the next day.

3- to 4-pound young chicken
1 cup bottled teriyaki marinade

1. Place chicken in a large zip-top plastic bag, add the marinade, and place in the refrigerator for 24 hours (flip bag over once or twice during this time, to let all of the chicken meat come in contact with the marinade).
2. After marinating, remove chicken from the bag and let excess marinade drip off (there will be a lot of excess to discard). Place chicken in the slow cooker crock, breast-side down.
3. Cover and cook on LOW for 6 hours; check for doneness using an instant-read thermometer (it should register 170°F). When done, let the bird rest in the crock, uncovered, for 5 minutes before serving.

approximate nutritional content
   ▶ Calories: 579, Protein: 82g, Net Carbs: 10g, Fat: 21g, Cholesterol: 253mg, Sodium: 753mg

▶ **cook's tip**
Stock up on young chickens when they're on special at the supermarket. We've seen them for as little as $0.69 a pound! Freeze them in large freezer bags until you need them.

▶ **about the ingredients**
Although some teriyaki marinades can be quite high in carbs, most of it is discarded in this recipe. Experiment with other bottled marinades to find your favorite.

sofrito chicken

▶ **ESTIMATED PREPARATION TIME:** 5 minutes   ▶ **COOK TIME:** 8 hours   ▶ **SERVINGS:** 4

This easy dish delivers full flavors with a minimum of fuss. Just the thing for a busy weekday dinner.

2 tablespoons olive oil

⅔ cup prepared *sofrito*

2 tablespoons minced garlic

3 celery stalks, sliced thinly on the diagonal

¼ teaspoon kosher salt

½ teaspoon black pepper

2 pounds skinless, boneless chicken thighs, fat trimmed

1. Grease the slow cooker crock with olive oil (leave excess in the crock). Add all ingredients, except chicken thighs, to the slow cooker crock and mix well to combine.

2. Add the chicken thighs and toss to coat chicken with *sofrito* mixture. Cover and cook on LOW for 8 hours.

approximate nutritional content

▶ Calories: 486, Protein: 52g, Net Carbs: 9g, Fat: 29g, Cholesterol: 189mg, Sodium: 595mg

---

▶ **serving suggestion**

Super Delish Snap Peas (page 198) would make an excellent accompaniment to this dish.

▶ **about the ingredients**

Sofrito is a bottled seasoning mixture containing tomatoes, green peppers, onions, garlic, olives, and seasonings. It's an easy way to pump up the flavor in a variety of dishes. Look for it in the "ethnic" section of the grocery store; we used the Goya brand.

turkey and cheddar roll-ups with cream sauce

▶ **ESTIMATED PREPARATION TIME:** 15 minutes ▶ **COOK TIME:** 4 hours ▶ **SERVINGS:** 4

Easy, impressive, and delicious. Pop it into the slow cooker before an afternoon of errands and you'll have a lovely meal when you arrive back home.

2 pounds scallopine-style (thin) turkey cutlets

8 ounces reduced-fat sharp cheddar cheese, cut into 12 rectangular pieces

½ cup white wine

1 packet dry vegetable soup mix

½ teaspoon black pepper

¼ teaspoon Tabasco sauce (about 2 shakes)

¼ cup half-and-half

1. Working with one cutlet at a time, place one piece of cheese onto the short edge of a turkey cutlet, then roll up and place the roll-ups in the slow cooker crock. Repeat with remaining pieces of turkey and cheese.

2. In a small bowl, combine remaining ingredients, except for the half-and-half; mix well and pour mixture over the turkey rolls.

3. Cover and cook on LOW for 4 hours. When done, remove turkey roll-ups using tongs and place on a serving dish (or on individual dishes). Turn slow cooker to high, add the half-and-half to the cooking juices, and mix well with a whisk. Once the cream has heated through, turn off slow cooker and pour sauce over the turkey roll-ups.

approximate nutritional content
▶ Calories: 491, Protein: 67g, Net Carbs: 8g, Fat: 16g, Cholesterol: 192mg, Sodium: 1,321mg

---

▶ **serving suggestion**
Warm Asparagus and Red Pepper Salad (page 190) would be delicious with this dish.

---

cheeseburger soup

▶ **ESTIMATED PREPARATION TIME:** 5 minutes   ▶ **COOK TIME:** 4 hours   ▶ **SERVINGS:** 4

Nice and easy for a weekend "soup night," and kids really love it. It's like a cheeseburger in a bowl! —KB

1 pound lean ground beef (90% lean)

1 medium onion, halved and chopped

1 10.75-ounce can condensed cheddar cheese soup

1 cup beef broth

1 14.5-ounce can "petite" diced tomatoes or regular diced tomatoes (do not drain)

shredded cheddar cheese (optional)

1. In a medium skillet, over medium heat, brown the beef and onion until beef is cooked through; drain off the fat.
2. Combine the beef and onion mixture with the remaining ingredients in the slow cooker crock; stir well.
3. Cover and cook on LOW for 4 hours. Stir before serving, and garnish each serving with a sprinkle of shredded cheese, if desired.

approximate nutritional content
▶ Calories: 383, Protein: 31g, Net Carbs: 10g, Fat: 22g, Cholesterol: 104mg, Sodium: 1,183mg

---

▶ **serving suggestion**

For a tangy side dish, try Kim's Mom's Cucumber Salad (page 193).

---

pesto beef with grape tomatoes and fresh mozzarella

▶ **ESTIMATED PREPARATION TIME:** 10 minutes ▶ **COOK TIME:** 6 hours ▶ **SERVINGS:** 6

This dish makes a beautiful presentation that will "wow" your family and friends. Plus, it's easy!

1 tablespoon olive oil

2 teaspoons dried minced onion

½ cup prepared pesto sauce

½ teaspoon black pepper

2 pounds round steak, cut into six pieces

2 pints grape tomatoes (about 4½ cups)

1 pound fresh mozzarella, drained, sliced, and brought to room temperature by serving time

1. Grease the slow cooker crock with olive oil (leave excess in the crock). Add the onion, pesto, and pepper to the crock, and stir to combine.

2. Add the steak to the crock and turn the pieces with tongs to coat with the pesto mixture; add the tomatoes.

3. Cover and cook on LOW for 6 hours. To serve, use clean tongs to place steak in individual bowls. Top each serving with a couple of slices of mozzarella, and some of the tomato mixture (use a slotted spoon to get tomatoes out of the slow cooker). If you like, some of the cooking juices can be added to each bowl, as well.

approximate nutritional content
  ▶ Calories: 624, Protein: 62g, Net Carbs: 7g, Fat: 35g, Cholesterol: 171mg, Sodium: 634mg

EASY SUBSTITUTION

Not in the mood for beef? Substitute 2 pounds of skinless, boneless, chicken breasts for the beef in this recipe. This will alter the approximate nutritional content to:
  ▶ Calories: 604, Protein: 61g, Net Carbs: 7g, Fat: 33g, Cholesterol: 172mg, Sodium: 651mg

ham with cranberry and horseradish sauce

▶ **PREPARATION TIME:** 5 minutes   ▶ **COOKING TIME:** 7 hours   ▶ **SERVINGS:** 6

Super-easy, and a great dish to make for a casual supper with family and friends.

1 pound bag fresh or frozen cranberries, rinsed and picked over
1 cup Splenda Granular sweetener
1 cup water
1½ tablespoons prepared horseradish
pinch kosher salt
3-pound boneless ham

1. Add all ingredients except ham to the slow cooker crock and mix well. Place ham on top of the cranberry mixture.
2. Cover and cook on LOW for 7 hours, stirring sauce (around the ham) halfway through the cooking process. Some of the cranberries may pop during cooking or when you stir; that's okay.
3. When done cooking, let ham rest in the slow cooker, uncovered, for 10 minutes before slicing. Serve a large spoonful of the cranberry sauce alongside each serving of ham.

approximate nutritional content
▶ Calories: 380, Protein: 55g, Net Carbs: 7g, Fat: 12g, Cholesterol: 120mg, Sodium: 2,951mg

▶ **serving suggestion**
A relish tray with olives, pickles, raw vegetables, and dip is a nice way to start this meal. Serve with steamed cauliflower or our Green Beans with Bacon (page 201).

teriyaki steak with peppers and onions

▶ **ESTIMATED PREPARATION TIME:** 10 minutes (plus 24 hours marinating time)   ▶ **COOK TIME:** 8 hours   ▶ **SERVINGS:** 4

This delicious dish is easy to make, and utilizes an inexpensive cut of beef.

2 pounds top round or London broil steak, trimmed

$\frac{1}{2}$ cup plus 1 tablespoon bottled teriyaki marinade, divided

1 medium onion, thinly sliced

1 red bell pepper, thinly sliced

1 green bell pepper, thinly sliced

1. In a large zip-top plastic bag, combine $\frac{1}{2}$ cup of marinade and steak; refrigerate 24 hours.

2. After marinating, transfer steak (using tongs) from the bag to the slow cooker crock; discard remaining marinade. Add onions and peppers to the crock.

3. Cover and cook on LOW for 8 hours. When done, let everything rest in the slow cooker, uncovered, for 10 minutes. Using clean tongs, move steak to a cutting board and slice it thin.

4. Spoon out $\frac{1}{4}$ cup of the cooking liquid and discard it. Add the 1 tablespoon more of fresh marinade from the bottle to the juices in the slow cooker crock and stir. Place sliced steak back into the crock and toss with the onion and pepper mixture.

approximate nutritional content
▶ Calories: 452, Protein: 55g, Net Carbs: 9g, Fat: 20g, Cholesterol: 133mg, Sodium: 426m

EASY ADD-IN
If you like, add one 7-ounce can of sliced mushrooms (drained) to the pepper and onion slices. Doing so will alter the approximate nutritional content to:
▶ Calories: 463, Protein: 55g, Net Carbs: 10g, Fat: 20g, Cholesterol: 133mg, Sodium: 607mg

---

▶ **about the ingredients**

London broil is an inexpensive cut of beef that works well in slow cooker recipes. Marinating the beef is key: it not only adds flavor, it tenderizes the meat, too.

---

souvlaki pork cutlets

▶ **ESTIMATED PREPARATION TIME:** 10 minutes   ▶ **COOK TIME:** 8 hours, (plus overnight marinating time)   ▶ **SERVINGS:** 4

This is super-fast if you prep the ingredients the night before, then just toss them into the slow cooker the next morning on your way out—don't forget to turn on the slow cooker, though!

2 pounds boneless pork sirloin cutlets

1½ teaspoon kosher salt

1½ teaspoon black pepper

6 cloves fresh garlic, minced

¼ cup olive oil

½ teaspoon Splenda Granular sweetener

½ cup water

1 lemon, cut in half

1. Place the pork in a large zip-top bag; set aside.
2. In a small mixing bowl, stir together the remaining ingredients, except for the lemon halves. Squeeze the juice from the lemon halves (save the juiced halves) into the mixing bowl and stir to combine. Pour the mixture into the zip-top bag, and add the two lemon halves. Shake the bag gently to make sure the meat is coated with the mixture, then place it in the refrigerator overnight.
3. The next morning, pour everything into the slow cooker (the pork and the marinating liquid and lemons). Cover and cook on LOW for 8 hours.
4. Before serving, remove lemon halves and stir.

approximate nutritional content
  ▶ Calories: 520, Protein: 54g, Net Carbs: 2g, Fat: 31g, Cholesterol: 160mg, Sodium: 286mg

EASY SUBSTITUTION

No pork on hand? Substitute 2 pounds of skinless, boneless chicken thighs. Doing so will alter the approximate nutritional content to:
  ▶ Calories: 486, Protein: 45g, Net Carbs: 2g, Fat: 32g, Cholesterol: 162mg, Sodium: 331mg

> ▶ **serving suggestion**
> This dish tastes great when paired with Broccoli Rabe with Pine Nuts (page 203), or chopped tomatoes topped with Cucumber-Yogurt Dressing (page 184).

mixed sausage with fennel

▶ **ESTIMATED PREPARATION TIME:** 10 minutes ▶ **COOK TIME:** 8 hours ▶ **SERVINGS:** 6

This is a unique and hearty dish to serve guests on a chilly fall or winter night. Feel free to use whatever type of sausage you prefer.

cooking spray

3 fennel bulbs, tops and bottoms removed, sliced into $\frac{1}{4}$-inch pieces

1 medium onion, halved and thinly sliced

$\frac{1}{4}$ teaspoon kosher salt

$\frac{1}{4}$ teaspoon black pepper

2 tablespoons water

2 pounds mixed sausages, cut in half crosswise

$\frac{1}{4}$ cup grated Parmesan cheese

1. Coat the slow cooker crock with cooking spray. Add the fennel, onion, salt, pepper, and water; toss to combine. Top with the sausage pieces.
2. Cover and cook on LOW for 8 hours.
3. To serve, place sausage pieces on top of some of the fennel in individual bowls, then sprinkle each serving with a little Parmesan cheese.

approximate nutritional content

▶ Calories: 561, Protein: 24g, Net Carbs: 3.5g, Fat: 49g, Cholesterol: 118mg, Sodium: 1,228mg

sausage with chickpeas and tomatoes

▶ **ESTIMATED PREPARATION TIME:** 5 minutes   ▶ **COOK TIME:** 8 hours   ▶ **SERVINGS:** 6

One taste and you'll think you're in Italy…

2 tablespoons tomato paste

2 tablespoons minced garlic

1 14.5-ounce can diced tomatoes

1 teaspoon dried rosemary

$\frac{1}{8}$ teaspoon kosher salt

1 teaspoon black pepper

1 15.5-ounce can chickpeas, drained

2 pounds Italian sausage, cut in half cross-wise

1. Add all ingredients except the chickpeas and sausage to the slow cooker crock; stir well.
2. Sprinkle chickpeas over the mixture, then top with sausage. Cover and cook on LOW for 8 hours.

approximate nutritional content

▶ Calories: 596, Protein: 25g, Net Carbs: 11g, Fat: 49g, Cholesterol: 115mg, Sodium: 1,443mg

EASY SUBSTITUTION

If you like, substitute 2 pounds of chicken tenders for the sausage. However, you'll need to mix them into the tomato mixture to coat them, then sprinkle the chickpeas on top. Also, you'll need an additional $\frac{1}{2}$ teaspoon of salt to make up for the seasoning that the sausage provides. The approximate nutritional content of this variation is:

▶ Calories: 291, Protein: 45g, Net Carbs: 10g, Fat: 6g, Cholesterol: 112mg, Sodium: 463mg

> ▶ **serving suggestion**
> A nice complement to these flavors would be our Broccoli Rabe with Pine Nuts (page 203).

italian sausage and peppers

▶ **ESTIMATED PREPARATION TIME:** 10 minutes   ▶ **COOK TIME:** 8 hours   ▶ **SERVINGS:** 6

This classic combination doesn't get much easier! For crisp vegetables, add the peppers and onions halfway through cooking, being sure to stir them in with the sausages.

2 pounds Italian sausage, cut in half
    crosswise

3 bell peppers, sliced into $\frac{1}{2}$-inch strips

2 medium onions, halved and thinly sliced

1 teaspoon black pepper

$\frac{1}{2}$ teaspoon kosher salt

2 teaspoons olive oil

sour cream (optional)

1. Add all ingredients to the slow cooker crock and toss well to coat vegetables and sausage pieces with the oil and spices.

2. Cover and cook on LOW for 8 hours. Garnish each serving with a dollop of sour cream, if desired.

approximate nutritional content
▶ Calories: 555, Protein: 22g, Net Carbs: 4g, Fat: 49g, Cholesterol: 115mg, Sodium: 1,147mg

EASY ADD-IN
If you're a mushroom lover, feel free to add a 7-ounce can of sliced mushrooms (drained) to the recipe. Doing so will alter the approximate nutritional content to:
▶ Calories: 564, Protein: 23g, Net Carbs: 5.5g, Fat: 49g, Cholesterol: 115mg, Sodium: 1,149mg

> ▶ **cook's tip**
> The sausages will not brown in the slow cooker. If you want them browned, sear them in a hot pan before adding to the slow cooker.

kielbasa, cabbage, and onions

▶ **PREPARATION TIME:** 5 minutes ▶ **COOKING TIME:** 8 hours ▶ **SERVINGS:** 6

These flavors may remind you of something your grandmother used to cook. A great dish for a simple fall supper.

cooking spray
1 small head of cabbage, cored and cut into wedges (about 2½ pounds)
1 medium onion, halved and thinly sliced
½ teaspoon kosher salt
½ teaspoon black pepper
2 cups chicken broth
2 tablespoons brown mustard
2 pounds kielbasa (or "lite" kielbasa, if you prefer), cut into 3-inch pieces

1. Coat the slow cooker crock with cooking spray. Add all ingredients except the kielbasa to the crock, tossing so that the cabbage is well-coated with the broth and seasonings. Top mixture with the kielbasa.
2. Cover and cook on LOW for 7 hours; give mixture a good stir, then cook 1 hour more.

approximate nutritional content
▶ Calories: 541, Protein: 24g, Net Carbs: 11g, Fat: 43g, Cholesterol: 103mg, Sodium: 2,162mg

▶ **serving suggestion**
Serve this dish with toasted, buttered, low-carb rye bread. If desired, pass malt vinegar and butter to season the cabbage.

tapenade swordfish with tomato sauce

▶ **PREPARATION TIME:** 10 minutes ▶ **COOKING TIME:** 4 hours ▶ **SERVINGS:** 4

So elegant, and no one needs to know it only took a few minutes to put together.

1 8-ounce can tomato sauce

¼ teaspoon kosher salt

½ teaspoon black pepper

⅓ cup ready-made tapenade

2 pounds swordfish steaks, skin removed

1. Stir together the tomato sauce, salt, and pepper in the slow cooker crock; set aside.
2. Spread tapenade evenly over one side of the swordfish steaks. Place swordfish, tapenade-side up, into the tomato sauce mixture.
3. Cover and cook on LOW for 4 hours. Using a spatula, transfer swordfish steaks to individual plates. Stir the sauce to combine, then ladle alongside the swordfish.

approximate nutritional content
   ▶ Calories: 363, Protein: 52g, Net Carbs: 4g, Fat: 13g, Cholesterol: 105mg, Sodium: 756mg

EASY SUBSTITUTION

If you're not a fish fan, feel free to substitute 2 pounds of skinless, boneless chicken breast for the swordfish. Doing so will change the approximate nutritional content to:
   ▶ Calories: 387, Protein: 64g, Net Carbs: 4g, Fat: 10g, Cholesterol: 176mg, Sodium: 700mg

> ▶ **about the ingredients**
> Tapenade, a purée of anchovies, garlic, black olives, and capers (and sometimes additional ingredients such as feta cheese), is sometimes found near the refrigerated hummus in the grocery store, or in the Italian foods section.

mediterranean hake

▶ **PREPARATION TIME:** 10 minutes ▶ **COOKING TIME:** 4 hours ▶ **SERVINGS:** 4

This easy recipe has great flavor and is a good way to get some fish into your diet if you're not a big fish lover. Hake is widely available, and its mild flavor is very pleasing when combined with the tomatoes and olives. —KB

1 28-ounce can of diced tomatoes with oregano, basil and garlic
16 small pimento-stuffed olives
1 tablespoon olive oil
1 teaspoon minced garlic
2 pounds hake fillet, cut into bite-sized pieces
shredded Parmesan cheese (optional)

1. Mix together all ingredients, except for the hake, in the slow cooker crock. Place the hake pieces on top of the tomato mixture.
2. Cover and cook on LOW for 4 hours. Stir well before serving, then ladle into individual bowls and top with a sprinkle of shredded Parmesan, if desired.

approximate nutritional content
▶ Calories: 370, Protein: 51g, Net Carbs: 9g, Fat: 12g, Cholesterol: 134mg, Sodium: 1,432mg

▶ **cook's tip**
If you can't find hake, substitute Atlantic wolf fish.

▶ **serving suggestion**
Our Sautéed Baby Spinach (page 200) makes an excellent addition to this dish.

soups, stews, and chilies

chicken soup

▶ **PREPARATION TIME:** 15 minutes ▶ **COOKING TIME:** 8 hours ▶ **SERVINGS:** 6

An all-time favorite made easier because of the slow cooker. Be sure to try the variations, too!

1 medium onion, finely chopped

4 celery stalks, finely chopped

3 carrots, peeled and finely chopped

1 tablespoon minced garlic

½ teaspoon kosher salt

1 teaspoon black pepper

2 pounds cooked chicken breast, cut into bite-sized pieces (about 4 cups)

2 tablespoons butter

3 14.5-ounce cans chicken broth

2 cubes chicken bouillon

¼ cup finely chopped fresh parsley

¼ teaspoon Tabasco sauce (about 2 shakes)

1. Place the vegetables, garlic, salt, and pepper in the slow cooker crock. Top with the chicken pieces, butter, broth, and bouillon. Do NOT stir.
2. Cover and cook on LOW for 8 hours.
3. Before serving, stir in parsley and Tabasco sauce.

approximate nutritional content
▶ Calories: 350, Protein: 49g, Net Carbs: 5g, Fat: 13g, Cholesterol: 143mg, Sodium: 1,484mg

EASY ADD-IN

If you like your chicken soup with noodles, feel free to add in 1½ cups low-carb, uncooked spaghetti, broken into pieces, to the soup during the last ½ hour of cooking. Doing so will change the approximate nutritional content to:
▶ Calories: 404, Protein: 58g, Net Carbs: 9g, Fat: 13g, Cholesterol: 143mg, Sodium: 1,498mg

EASY SUBSTITUTIONS

If you don't have cooked chicken meat handy, you can either microwave raw chicken breast or add uncooked chicken to the crock. However, the uncooked chicken will make the soup broth cloudy instead of clear.

Feel free to substitute cooked turkey meat instead of the chicken. Handy after Thanksgiving!

chicken-barley soup

▶ **PREPARATION TIME:** 15 minutes ▶ **COOKING TIME:** 8 hours ▶ **SERVINGS:** 6

Our chicken soup recipe (page 52) gets a boost of grains in this hearty version.

1 medium onion, finely chopped

4 celery stalks, finely chopped

3 carrots, peeled and finely chopped

1 tablespoon minced garlic

½ teaspoon kosher salt

1 teaspoon black pepper

2 pounds cooked chicken breast, cut into
     bite-sized pieces (about 4 cups)

½ cup barley, picked over and rinsed

2 tablespoons butter

3 14.5-ounce cans chicken broth

1 cup water

2 cubes chicken bouillon

¼ cup finely chopped fresh parsley

¼ teaspoon Tabasco sauce (about 2
     shakes)

1. Place the vegetables, garlic, salt, and pepper in the slow cooker crock. Top with chicken pieces, barley, butter, broth, water, and bouillon. Do NOT stir.

2. Cover and cook on LOW for 8 hours.

3. Before serving, stir in parsley and Tabasco sauce.

approximate nutritional content
▶ Calories: 405, Protein: 51g, Net Carbs: 14g, Fat: 13g, Cholesterol: 143mg, Sodium: 1,486mg

soups, stews, and chilies **53**

chicken, tomato, and white bean soup

▶ **PREPARATION TIME:** 15 minutes   ▶ **COOKING TIME:** 8 hours   ▶ **SERVINGS:** 6

Even more vegetables makes this version of our Chicken Soup recipe (page 52) especially tasty and filling!

1 medium onion, finely chopped

4 celery stalks, finely chopped

3 carrots, peeled and finely chopped

1 tablespoon minced garlic

½ teaspoon kosher salt

1 teaspoon black pepper

2 pounds cooked chicken breast, cut into bite-sized pieces (about 4 cups)

2 tablespoons butter

3 14.5-ounce cans chicken broth

2 cubes chicken bouillon

1 14.5-ounce can diced tomatoes, drained

1 14.5-ounce can white beans, drained and rinsed

¼ cup finely chopped fresh parsley

¼ teaspoon Tabasco sauce (about 2 shakes)

1. Place the vegetables, garlic, salt, and pepper in the slow cooker crock. Top with the chicken pieces, butter, broth, and bouillon. Do NOT stir.
2. Cover and cook on LOW for 7½ hours. Stir in drained tomatoes and beans; continue to cook ½ hour more.
3. Before serving, stir in parsley and Tabasco sauce.

approximate nutritional content

▶ Calories: 410, Protein: 52g, Net Carbs: 13g, Fat: 13g, Cholesterol: 143mg, Sodium: 1,712mg

dude ranch soup

▶ **ESTIMATED PREPARATION TIME:** 10 minutes   ▶ **COOK TIME:** 8 hours   ▶ **SERVINGS:** 6

Obviously, my husband named this soup! It's a manly meal, but we little ladies enjoy it, too. —KM

2 pounds round steak, cut into bite-sized pieces

1 15.5-ounce can kidney beans, drained

1 4-ounce can chopped green chilies

3 celery stalks, finely chopped

1 14.5-ounce can beef broth

1 tablespoon tomato paste

1 teaspoon chili powder

1 teaspoon adobo seasoning

1 cube beef bouillon

1 teaspoon black pepper

1 teaspoon cumin

1 teaspoon minced garlic

3 tablespoons dried minced onions

1 cup reduced-fat shredded cheddar cheese

1. Add all ingredients except the cheese to the slow cooker crock and mix well.
2. Cover and cook on LOW for 7½ hours. Stir in cheddar cheese and cook ½ hour more.

approximate nutritional content
▶ Calories: 398, Protein: 53g, Net Carbs: 11.5g, Fat: 11g, Cholesterol: 125mg, Sodium: 1,024mg

▶ **about the ingredients**
Adobo seasoning is found at most supermarkets either in the "ethnic" aisle or the seasoning section; we used the Goya brand.

▶ **serving suggestion**
Our Zippy Coleslaw (page 194) would be great with this soup.

stuffed cabbage soup

▶ **ESTIMATED PREPARATION TIME:** 15 minutes ▶ **COOK TIME:** 10 hours ▶ **SERVINGS:** 6

This recipe is great when you want the flavors of authentic stuffed cabbage—without the fuss. We've substituted barley for rice to help keep the carbs down.

1 tablespoon olive oil

1½ pounds lean ground beef (90% lean)

1 medium onion, finely chopped

1 28-ounce can crushed tomatoes

2 cubes beef bouillon

⅓ cup barley, rinsed and picked over

2 teaspoons Splenda Granular sweetener

1 tablespoon minced garlic

1 teaspoon black pepper

¼ teaspoon Tabasco sauce (about 2 shakes)

½ head cabbage (about 1½ pounds), chopped

3 14.5-ounce cans beef broth

1. In a medium stock pot, over medium heat, warm the oil. Add beef and onion; cook until onions are soft and meat is browned throughout; about 8 minutes. Drain the fat off the meat mixture and add the tomatoes, bouillon, barley, Splenda, garlic, pepper, and Tabasco to the beef; mix all ingredients well and set aside.

2. Place the chopped cabbage in the slow cooker crock. Top with the reserved beef mixture; do not stir. Add the beef broth; do not stir.

3. Cover and cook on LOW 9 hours; stir the soup well, then re-cover and continue to cook 1 hour more.

approximate nutritional content
▶ Calories: 375, Protein: 36g, Net Carbs: 13g, Fat: 18g, Cholesterol: 101mg, Sodium: 1,457mg

▶ **serving suggestion**
For a nice and easy winter supper, serve the soup with slices of low-carb, buttered rye toast.

sausage and white bean soup

▸ **PREPARATION TIME:** 15 minutes ▸ **COOKING TIME:** 8 hours ▸ **SERVINGS:** 6

This is my husband's all-time favorite soup. It's also a great way to sneak some healthy greens into the guy's diet. —KM

1 tablespoon olive oil

2 pounds sweet Italian sausage, meat pushed out of casings

1 medium onion, finely chopped

1 tablespoon minced garlic

1 14.5-ounce can cannellini beans, drained

2 tablespoons tomato paste

1 teaspoon black pepper

1 tablespoon quick-cooking tapioca

1 14.5-ounce can chicken broth

1 head escarole, washed and chopped into bite-sized pieces

⅓ cup grated Parmesan cheese

1. In a large skillet, over medium heat, warm olive oil; add sausage meat and onions; cook until sausage is browned and onions are soft, about 7 minutes. Drain off any fat.

2. Add sausage and onion mixture to the slow cooker crock, then add all remaining ingredients, except escarole and Parmesan. Mix gently until tomato paste dissolves.

3. Cover and cook on LOW for 7 hours. Add chopped escarole; stir well and cook 1 hour more. Serve in individual bowls, topped with grated Parmesan cheese.

approximate nutritional content
▸ Calories: 489, Protein: 28g, Net Carbs: 12g, Fat: 34g, Cholesterol: 94mg, Sodium: 1,600mg

french onion soup

▶ **PREPARATION TIME:** 15 minutes   ▶ **COOKING TIME:** 8 hours   ▶ **SERVINGS:** 6

Nothing tastes — or smells—better than French Onion Soup topped with a crouton and melted cheese. You'll say "magnifique!" —KM

4 tablespoons butter

5 medium onions, halved and thinly sliced

½ teaspoon kosher salt

5 cups good-quality beef broth

½ teaspoon thyme

1 teaspoon black pepper

½ cup dry sherry

6 Giant Soup Croutons (page 183)

⅓ pound sliced Swiss or Gruyère cheese, at room temperature

1. In a medium skillet, over medium heat, melt butter. Add onions and sauté them with the salt until onions are soft and browned, about 10 minutes.

2. Add all ingredients, except the Giant Soup Croutons and cheese, to the slow cooker and mix well. Cover and cook on LOW for 7 hours. Stir well, then cook 1 hour more.

3. To serve, ladle soup into bowls, filling about ¾ full. Top with one of the Giant Soup Croutons and some of the cheese, then a little more soup, to melt the cheese. You may need to microwave the bowls for about 45 seconds to completely melt the cheese. To present the soup in restaurant fashion, ladle it into oven-proof bowls, then top with the croutons and cheese, and broil briefly until cheese is melted and lightly browned.

approximate nutritional content
Calories: 237, Protein: 12g, Net Carbs: 7g, Fat: 16g, Cholesterol: ▶ 45mg, Sodium: 1,045mg

▶ **serving suggestion**

A bowl of this soup, along with a simple green salad topped with a few toasted nuts, makes a perfect dinner.

vegetable and bean soup

▶ **PREPARATION TIME:** 20 minutes ▶ **COOKING TIME:** 8 hours ▶ **SERVINGS:** 6

Soup is one of my favorite ways to eat vegetables. I make a batch of this soup about once a month and freeze individual portions for lunches. —KM

1 14.5-ounce can diced tomatoes

2 14.5-ounce cans chicken broth

1 cube vegetable bouillon

1 medium onion, finely chopped

1 15.5-ounce can kidney beans, drained (or other favorite bean)

1 red bell pepper, finely chopped

2 carrots, finely chopped

2 celery stalks, finely chopped

2 summer squashes (zucchini or yellow squash, about 1 pound total), quartered lengthwise and chopped

1 7-ounce can sliced mushrooms, drained

1 tablespoon minced garlic

1 tablespoon olive oil

2 tablespoons butter

¼ teaspoon kosher salt

1 teaspoon black pepper

½ teaspoon Tabasco sauce (about 4 shakes) (optional)

1. Combine all ingredients in the slow cooker crock and mix well.
2. Cover and cook on LOW for 8 hours. Stir well before serving. If desired, stir in Tabasco sauce before serving.

approximate nutritional content

▶ Calories: 210, Protein: 8g, Net Carbs: 18g, Fat: 9g, Cholesterol: 14mg, Sodium: 1,020mg

EASY SUBSTITUTION

To make this soup completely vegetarian, substitute vegetable broth for the chicken broth, and additional olive oil for the butter.

▶ **serving suggestion**

Once you've ladled the soup into individual bowls, try garnishing it with a slice of fresh mozzarella or provolone cheese. Or, do as the Italians do and sprinkle on some Parmesan cheese. The heat of the soup melts the cheese and provides richness and flavor.

beef and vegetable stew

▶ **ESTIMATED PREPARATION TIME:** 15 minutes   ▶ **COOK TIME:** 8 hours   ▶ **SERVINGS:** 6

Searing the meat in hot oil and sautéing the vegetables creates a deeply flavored stew (you won't even miss the traditional potatoes). However, if you're in a hurry, eliminate Step 2 and simply stir in the beef and vegetables after Step 3.

cooking spray

¼ cup olive oil

2 pounds beef stew meat, fat trimmed

2 teaspoons minced garlic

2 medium onions, chopped

2 large carrots, peeled and cut into ¼-inch-thick "coins"

3 large celery stalks, sliced in half lengthwise and cut into ¼-inch pieces

1 teaspoon kosher salt

½ teaspoon black pepper

8 ounces mushrooms, quartered

14-ounce can diced tomatoes (undrained)

½ cup beef broth

2 tablespoons red wine

2 teaspoons Worcestershire sauce

1½ teaspoons ground thyme

1 bay leaf

1 tablespoon quick-cooking tapioca

1. Coat the inside of the slow cooker crock with cooking spray; set aside.
2. In a large skillet, over medium heat, warm the olive oil. Add beef and garlic; brown them approximately 4 minutes, then remove from heat and place mixture in the slow cooker crock.
3. Return the pan to the heat, add the onions, carrots, celery, salt, and pepper and cook until onions are softened, approximately 4 minutes; set aside.
4. To the slow cooker crock, add the mushrooms, tomatoes, beef broth, wine, Worcestershire sauce, thyme, bay leaf, and tapioca; stir until well-combined.
5. Add the reserved vegetables and stir to combine all ingredients. Cover and cook on LOW for 7 hours. Stir the stew, then cook 1 hour more. Before serving, remove bay leaf.

approximate nutritional content
▶ Calories: 486, Protein: 34g, Net Carbs: 10g, Fat: 33g, Cholesterol: 113mg, Sodium: 651mg

beef, bean, and bacon stew

▶ **ESTIMATED PREPARATION TIME:** 15 minutes ▶ **COOK TIME:** 8 hours ▶ **SERVINGS:** 6

In this variation of Beef and Vegetable Stew (page 60), the beans and bacon provide a unique flavor twist. For a smokier-tasting stew, choose a higher-quality, stronger-flavored bacon.

cooking spray

$\frac{1}{4}$ cup olive oil

2 pounds beef stew meat, fat trimmed

2 teaspoons minced garlic

2 medium onions, chopped

2 large carrots, peeled and cut into $\frac{1}{4}$-inch-thick "coins"

2 large celery stalks, sliced in half lengthwise and cut into $\frac{1}{4}$-inch pieces

1 teaspoon kosher salt

$\frac{1}{2}$ teaspoon black pepper

1 14.5 ounce-can diced tomatoes (undrained)

$\frac{1}{2}$ cup beef broth

2 tablespoons red wine

2 teaspoons Worcestershire sauce

$1\frac{1}{2}$ teaspoons ground thyme

1 bay leaf

1 tablespoon quick-cooking tapioca

$\frac{3}{4}$ cup canned kidney beans, drained and rinsed

2 slices bacon, cooked and roughly chopped

1. Coat the inside of the slow cooker crock with cooking spray; set aside.

2. In a large skillet, over medium heat, warm the olive oil. Add beef and garlic; brown them approximately 4 minutes, then remove from heat and place mixture in the slow cooker crock.

3. Return the pan to the heat, add the onions, carrots, celery, salt, and pepper and cook until onions are softened, approximately 4 minutes; set aside.

4. To the slow cooker crock, add the tomatoes, beef broth, wine, Worcestershire sauce, thyme, bay leaf, and tapioca; stir until well-combined.

5. Add the reserved vegetables and stir to combine all ingredients. Cover and cook on LOW for 7 hours. Stir in the kidney beans and bacon, then cook 1 hour more. Before serving, remove bay leaf.

approximate nutritional content
▶ Calories: 515, Protein: 36g, Net Carbs: 11.5g, Fat: 34g, Cholesterol: 115mg, Sodium: 748mg

pepper and onion beef stew

▶ **ESTIMATED PREPARATION TIME:** 10 minutes   ▶ **COOK TIME:** 10 hours   ▶ **SERVINGS:** 6

One of my favorite recipes in the whole book; it's fabulous and super-easy! Be sure
to serve it with Cheesy Mock Mashed Potatoes (page 170). —KB

1 tablespoon olive oil
1 tablespoon oregano
1 cup beef broth
1 cube beef bouillon
½ teaspoon celery salt
1 tablespoon Worcestershire sauce
1 tablespoon minced garlic
2 teaspoons soy sauce
2 tablespoons quick-cooking tapioca
2 tablespoons red wine
¼ teaspoon black pepper
2 green bell peppers, chopped
2 medium onions, chopped
2 pounds beef stew meat, fat trimmed
½ teaspoon crushed red pepper flakes
   (optional)

1. Add all ingredients to the slow cooker crock, stirring to
    mix well.
2. Cover and cook on LOW for 10 hours, stirring once
    during cooking.

approximate nutritional content
   ▶ Calories: 466, Protein: 38g, Net Carbs: 7.5g, Fat: 30g,
   Cholesterol: 132mg, Sodium: 1,021mg

EASY SUBSTITUTION

To add more color to the stew, substitute a red bell pepper for one of the
green ones.

beef and barley stew

▶ **ESTIMATED PREPARATION TIME:** 15 minutes ▶ **COOK TIME:** 8 hours ▶ **SERVINGS:** 6

No need to precook the meat with this one; it's truly a throw-it-all-in-the-pot-and-close-the-lid recipe. Nothing's better on a cold day than a hot bowl of this stew.

2 14.5-ounce cans of beef broth

2 tablespoons tomato paste

2 pounds beef stew meat, fat trimmed, cut into bite-sized pieces

1 8-ounce package sliced white mushrooms

½ medium onion, finely chopped

½ cup barley, rinsed and picked over

2 carrots, peeled and finely chopped

2 celery stalks, finely chopped

2 tablespoons butter

½ teaspoon thyme

¼ teaspoon rosemary

¼ teaspoon kosher salt

½ teaspoon black pepper

1 cube beef bouillon

1. Combine beef broth and tomato paste in the slow cooker crock; mix well. Add all remaining ingredients and stir to combine.

2. Cover and cook on LOW for 7 hours. Stir the stew well, then cook 1 hour more.

approximate nutritional content
   ▶ Calories: 446, Protein: 47g, Net Carbs: 14g, Fat: 20g, Cholesterol: 145mg, Sodium: 1,259mg

EASY ADD-IN

If you're a bacon lover, feel free to add ¼ cup chopped cooked bacon to this recipe for a nice smoky taste. Doing so will alter the approximate nutrition content to:
   ▶ Calories: 464, Protein: 48g, Net Carbs: 14g, Fat: 21g, Cholesterol: 147mg, Sodium: 1,309mg

▶ **about the ingredients**

Do not use pearl or quick-cooking barley in this recipe. This is the perfect opportunity to take advantage of what the slow cooker does best—create rich, wholesome dishes through long, slow cooking.

beef stew with chickpeas and spinach

▶ **PREPARATION TIME:** 15 minutes ▶ **COOK TIME:** 8 hours ▶ **SERVINGS:** 6

Hearty, rich, and very filling—a perfect winter night's meal.

¼ cup olive oil, divided

2 pounds beef stew meat, fat trimmed

1 medium onion, finely chopped

¼ teaspoon kosher salt

1 14.5-ounce can chickpeas, drained

1 10-ounce package frozen chopped spinach, thawed and water pressed out

¼ cup tomato paste

1 teaspoon black pepper

¼ teaspoon Splenda Granular sweetener

1 cube beef bouillon

2½ cups water

1. Use 1 tablespoon of the olive oil to grease the slow cooker crock; set aside.

2. Heat remaining olive oil in a large skillet over medium heat. Add beef, onion, and salt to the pan and brown the meat about 8 minutes, until cooked through and onions are soft; drain any liquid and set aside.

3. Add chickpeas, spinach, tomato paste, pepper, Splenda, bouillon, and water to the slow cooker; mix to dissolve the tomato paste. Add beef mixture and stir to combine. Cover and cook on LOW for 8 hours.

approximate nutritional content
▶ Calories: 602, Protein: 44g, Net Carbs: 16g, Fat: 38g, Cholesterol: 415mg, Sodium: 676mg

beef and sausage stew

▶ **ESTIMATED PREPARATION TIME:** 15 minutes ▶ **COOK TIME:** 8 hours ▶ **SERVINGS:** 6

A meat lover's dream: The combination of beef, sausage, and vegetables makes
this a very hearty, delicious stew—it's super-easy, too!

1 tablespoon olive oil

1 pound Italian sausage links (sweet or hot), meat pushed out of casings

1 pound beef stew meat, fat trimmed

1 14.5-ounce can beef broth

2 tablespoons tomato paste

1 10-ounce package white mushrooms, quartered

2 celery stalks, sliced thinly

2 cubes beef bouillon

1 teaspoon black pepper

1 teaspoon oregano

1 head cauliflower, halved, cored, and cut into bite-sized pieces (about 4 cups)

1 tablespoon minced garlic

1 tablespoon Worcestershire sauce

½ teaspoon Tabasco sauce (about 4 shakes)

1. In a skillet over medium heat, warm olive oil; brown sausage and stew meat until thoroughly cooked; drain off fat and set aside.

2. Whisk together the beef broth and tomato paste in the slow cooker crock. Add all remaining ingredients, as well as cooked sausage and stew meat, and stir together.

3. Cover and cook on LOW for 8 hours. Stir well before serving.

approximate nutritional content
▶ Calories: 365, Protein: 33g, Net Carbs: 7g, Fat: 22g, Cholesterol: 102mg, Sodium: 1,377mg

middle eastern chicken, lentil, and spinach stew

▶ **PREPARATION TIME:** 10 minutes   ▶ **COOKING TIME:** 6 hours   ▶ **SERVINGS:** 5

This dish is sure to break up your dinner doldrums! Plus, it's a meal-in-a-pot—whole grains, vegetables, and protein.

2 tablespoons olive oil

2 pounds skinless, boneless chicken breast, fat trimmed, cut into bite-sized pieces

1 10-ounce package frozen chopped spinach, thawed and water pressed out

1 medium onion, finely chopped

1 carrot, finely chopped

¾ cup lentils, rinsed and picked over

2 cups chicken broth

½ lemon

½ cup water

1. Grease the slow cooker crock with the olive oil (leave excess in the crock). Add all remaining ingredients, except for the lemon and water; mix well.

2. Push the lemon, cut–side down, into the middle of the mixture.

3. Cover and cook on LOW for 6 hours. When done, add the water and mix well before serving.

approximate nutritional content
▶ Calories: 457, Protein: 60g, Net Carbs: 19g, Fat: 13g, Cholesterol: 137mg, Sodium: 623mg

good ol' chili

▶ **ESTIMATED PREPARATION TIME:** 15 minutes ▶ **COOK TIME:** 8 hours ▶ **SERVINGS:** 6

This is your typical chili, revamped for low-carb dieters. Perfect for soup night or football Sundays—serve with a few low-carb tortilla chips, guacamole, and low-carb beer.

1 tablespoon vegetable oil

2 pounds lean ground beef (90% lean)

1 medium onion, chopped

1 teaspoon black pepper

1 teaspoon kosher salt

1 green bell pepper, chopped

1 14.5-ounce can kidney beans, drained

1 14.5-ounce can diced tomatoes with green chilies

1 14.5-ounce can beef broth

2 tablespoons chili powder

1 tablespoon minced garlic

2 teaspoons oregano

1 cube beef bouillon

1 teaspoon cumin

shredded cheddar cheese (optional)

Tabasco sauce (optional)

1. In a large skillet, over medium heat, warm oil; add beef, onion, pepper, and salt. Cook and stir until beef is broken up and cooked through. Drain fat and add beef mixture to the slow cooker crock.

2. Add all remaining ingredients, except for cheese and Tabasco sauce, to the slow cooker crock and stir to combine.

3. Cover and cook on LOW for 8 hours, stirring a few times during cooking. Stir well before serving. Offer shredded cheese and Tabasco sauce when serving.

approximate nutritional content

▶ Calories: 500, Protein: 47g, Net Carbs: 13g, Fat: 24g, Cholesterol: 142mg, Sodium: 898mg

EASY SUBSTITUTION

Substitute ground turkey for the ground beef. This will change the approximate nutritional content to:

▶ Calories: 357, Protein: 31g, Net Carbs: 13g, Fat: 17g, Cholesterol: 108mg, Sodium: 990mg

good ol' vegetarian chili

▶ **ESTIMATED PREPARATION TIME:** 15 minutes ▶ **COOK TIME:** 8 hours ▶ **SERVINGS:** 8

If you like chili but want to go meat-free, try this version of Good Ol' Chili (page 67). Note the higher carb level, due to the vegetable crumbles.

2 pounds frozen beef-flavored vegetarian crumbles

1 medium onion, chopped

1 teaspoon black pepper

1 teaspoon kosher salt

1 green bell pepper, chopped

1 14.5-ounce can kidney beans, drained

1 14.5-ounce can diced tomatoes with green chilies

1 14.5-ounce can vegetable broth

2 tablespoons chili powder

1 tablespoon minced garlic

2 teaspoons oregano

1 cube vegetable bouillon

1 teaspoon cumin

shredded cheddar cheese (optional)

Tabasco sauce (optional)

1. Add all ingredients except for the cheese and Tabasco sauce to the slow cooker crock; stir to combine.
2. Cover and cook on LOW for 8 hours, stirring a few times during cooking. Stir well before serving. Offer shredded cheese and Tabasco sauce when serving.

approximate nutritional content
▶ Calories: 314, Protein: 24g, Net Carbs: 23g, Fat: 12g, Cholesterol: 0mg, Sodium: 1,886mg

ciao bella chili

▶ **ESTIMATED PREPARATION TIME:** 15 minutes ▶ **COOK TIME:** 8 hours ▶ **SERVINGS:** 6

This is a fun twist on the traditional ground-beef-and-kidney-bean chili.

2 pounds Italian sausage (sweet or hot)

1 28-ounce can diced tomatoes

1 14.5-ounce can chickpeas, drained

1 tablespoon minced garlic

2 tablespoons dried minced onions

1 bay leaf

1 teaspoon black pepper

½ teaspoon crushed red pepper flakes

2 cups low-sodium chicken broth

fresh mozzarella or provolone cubes
   (optional)

1. Pierce each sausage link several times with a paring knife, then place in a medium stock pot and cover with water. Bring to a boil over medium–high heat; boil 10 minutes.

2. While sausages are boiling, add all remaining ingredients, except for cheese cubes, to the slow cooker crock.

3. Remove sausages from the boiling water and let cool slightly on a clean cutting board. Slice each sausage link in half lengthwise, then cut into "half-moons" about ¼-inch thick. Add sausage to the slow cooker crock and mix all ingredients well.

4. Cover and cook on LOW for 8 hours. Stir well before serving, and remove bay leaf. Garnish each portion with cheese cubes, if desired.

approximate nutritional content
   ▶ Calories: 515, Protein: 28g, Net Carbs: 14g, Fat: 37g, Cholesterol: 96mg, Sodium: 1,902mg

▶ **cook's tips**

▪ For easy morning preparation, boil the sausages the night before, then refrigerate them until the morning. The next morning, put everything right into the slow cooker and walk out the door!

▪ This dish tastes even better if it sits overnight in the refrigerator after cooking, plus this allows you to skim any unwanted fat off the surface before reheating it in your microwave.

soups, stews, and chilies **69**

texas chili

▸ **ESTIMATED PREPARATION TIME:** 5 minutes ▸ **COOK TIME:** 8 hours ▸ **SERVINGS:** 6

Texas chili is typically very spicy and contains no beans or tomatoes. We've toned down the spiciness a bit, in order to appeal to more people, but feel free to add more red pepper flakes if you really want to sweat!

3 pounds chuck beef stew meat, fat trimmed

1 tablespoon minced garlic

¼ cup chili powder

1 teaspoon red pepper flakes (or to taste)

2 tablespoons quick-cooking tapioca

1 tablespoon oregano

1 teaspoon cumin

2 cubes beef bouillon

1 teaspoon black pepper

1 14.5-ounce can beef broth

½ medium onion, finely chopped

sour cream (optional)

lime wedges (optional)

1. Add all ingredients to the slow cooker crock and mix well. Cover and cook on LOW for 8 hours.
2. Stir chili well before serving, and offer with sour cream and a wedge of lime, for a traditional Texas garnish.

approximate nutritional content
▸ Calories: 487, Protein: 61g, Net Carbs: 5.5g, Fat: 23g, Cholesterol: 192mg, Sodium: 1,193mg

---

▸ **serving suggestion**

Serve with our Creamy Coleslaw (page 195) or Faux Potato Salad (page 192).

▸ **cook's tip**

To make authentic Texas chili, you must use chuck beef. If your grocer doesn't offer chuck stew meat, ask the butcher to cut up a chuck shoulder roast for you.

white chili

▶ **ESTIMATED PREPARATION TIME:** 15 minutes ▶ **COOK TIME:** 8 hours ▶ **SERVINGS:** 6

Great for informal gatherings, this recipe lets you make one big pot from which guests can serve themselves, then sprinkle on their choice of toppings. Do not skip the first step, in which the turkey is precooked; putting raw turkey in the slow cooker results in a watery, unappetizing chili.

2 tablespoons vegetable oil

2 pounds ground turkey or ground chicken

1 medium onion, finely chopped

1 tablespoon minced garlic

1 teaspoon kosher salt

1½ cups chicken broth

1 tablespoon tomato paste

1 yellow bell pepper, chopped

1 tablespoon butter

¼ teaspoon red pepper flakes

1 teaspoon black pepper

1 teaspoon chili powder

1 teaspoon cumin

½ teaspoon Tabasco (about 4 shakes)

1 4-ounce can chopped green chilies, drained

1 19-ounce can great northern beans, drained

1. In a large skillet, over medium heat, warm the oil; add the turkey, onion, garlic, and salt and cook until the turkey is cooked through, breaking up the turkey as it cooks. Drain any remaining juices from the pan; set aside.

2. In the slow cooker crock, combine the broth and tomato paste and mix well. Add the turkey mixture to the crock, then add all remaining ingredients, except for the chilies and beans. Stir well to combine. Top with chilies and beans; do not stir again.

3. Cover and cook on LOW for 7 hours. Stir well, then cook 1 hour more.

approximate nutritional content
▶ Calories: 447, Protein: 39g, Net Carbs: 14g, Fat: 23g, Cholesterol: 122mg, Sodium: 555mg

> ▶ **serving suggestion**
> Serve this chili with do-it-yourself top-pings, such as sour cream, shredded cheddar cheese, and sliced scallions.

beef entrées

all-beef meatloaf

▶ **ESTIMATED PREPARATION TIME:** 10 minutes   ▶ **COOK TIME:** 8 hours   ▶ **SERVINGS:** 6

This recipe uses just a few simple ingredients and delivers a traditional, onion-flavored meatloaf. Be aware that low-carb meatloaf tends to be somewhat heavy because it doesn't have the benefit of regular (high-carb) bread. Luckily, it's also very moist. This one gets an extra flavor punch from the ketchup topping.

2 pounds lean ground beef (90% lean)
4 slices low-carb white bread, crusts discarded, and cut into ½-inch cubes
1 packet dry onion soup mix
½ teaspoon minced garlic
1 5.5-ounce can V8 juice
1 tablespoon Worcestershire sauce
2 eggs, beaten
½ medium onion, chopped
⅓ cup low-carb/low-sugar ketchup

1. In a large mixing bowl, combine all ingredients except for the ketchup. Mix well with clean hands to combine thoroughly.
2. Place the beef mixture into the slow cooker crock and form into a loaf shape. Cover and cook on LOW for 7 hours. Spoon ketchup over top of the loaf and cook 1 hour more.
3. Let loaf sit, uncovered, for 5 minutes, then transfer it to a serving plate, using a large spatula.

approximate nutritional content
▶ Calories: 459, Protein: 47g, Net Carbs: 6g, Fat: 24g, Cholesterol: 213mg, Sodium: 547mg

> ▶ **serving suggestion**
> This meatloaf is perfect with Cheesy Mock Mashed Potatoes (page 170) and a steamed green vegetable.

classic meatloaf

▶ **ESTIMATED PREPARATION TIME:** 10 minutes ▶ **COOK TIME:** 8 hours ▶ **SERVINGS:** 6

This may remind you of your mom's meatloaf! It calls for ground pork and ground veal, but feel free to use lean ground beef (90% lean) instead of veal, if you prefer.

1 8-ounce can tomato sauce

½ teaspoon Tabasco sauce (about 4 shakes)

3 eggs, beaten

2 slices of low-carb bread, crusts discarded, and cut into ½-inch cubes

1 pound ground pork

1 pound ground veal

¼ cup grated Parmesan cheese

2 teaspoons onion powder

1 teaspoon garlic powder

1 teaspoon kosher salt

1 teaspoon black pepper

1 teaspoon oregano

7 slices cooked bacon (not crispy)

1. In a large mixing bowl, combine tomato sauce, Tabasco, eggs, and bread cubes; let sit until bread absorbs the liquid, then blend well.

2. Mix in remaining ingredients, except for bacon, using clean hands. Place the mixture into the slow cooker crock and form into a loaf shape. Lay the bacon slices crosswise on top of the loaf, tucking the ends underneath the loaf.

3. Cover and cook on LOW for 8 hours. Let loaf sit, uncovered, for 5 minutes, then transfer it to a serving plate, using a large spatula.

approximate nutritional content
▶ Calories: 357, Protein: 41g, Net Carbs: 5g, Fat: 18g, Cholesterol: 223mg, Sodium: 659mg

---

▶ **serving suggestion**

This meatloaf is great with Summer Squash Sauté (page 199) or Creamy Coleslaw (page 195).

---

greek meatloaf

▶ **ESTIMATED PREPARATION TIME:** 5 minutes   ▶ **COOK TIME:** 8 hours   ▶ **SERVINGS:** 6

All the wonderful Greek flavors you love, in an easy-to-make, easy-to-serve loaf.

cooking spray
2 pounds lean ground beef (90% lean)
1 6-ounce package crumbled feta cheese
1 10-ounce package frozen chopped spinach (thawed and water pressed out)
3 eggs, beaten
2 teaspoons oregano
1 tablespoon minced garlic
1 teaspoon black pepper
1 tablespoon dried minced onions
¼ teaspoon red pepper flakes

1. Coat the slow cooker crock with cooking spray; set aside.
2. In a large mixing bowl, combine all ingredients and mix well. Transfer mixture to the slow cooker crock and form a loaf or a rounded mound shape.
3. Cover and cook on LOW for 8 hours. Let loaf sit, uncovered, for 5 minutes before serving.

approximate nutritional content
▶ Calories: 495, Protein: 50g, Net Carbs: 3g, Fat: 30g, Cholesterol: 273mg, Sodium: 455mg

---

▶ **serving suggestion**
Serve with chopped, fresh tomatoes, topped with Cucumber-Yogurt Dressing (page 184).

▶ **cook's tip**
Not sure if the meatloaf is seasoned appropriately for your family? A quick way to test it is to cook a small amount of the meat mixture in the microwave (or on the stove-top in a small frying pan) before forming the loaf. That way, you can taste-test your mixture, then add more seasoning, if desired.

mexican meatloaf

▶ **ESTIMATED PREPARATION TIME:** 5 minutes ▶ **COOK TIME:** 8 hours ▶ **SERVINGS:** 6

If you're craving the taste of tacos, this is your recipe!

cooking spray
2 pounds lean ground beef (90% lean)
1 14.5-ounce can of tomatoes with green chilies, drained
1 packet of taco seasoning
3 eggs, beaten
½ teaspoon black pepper
shredded "Mexican" blend cheese (optional)
sour cream (optional)
sliced scallions or chopped red onion (optional)
chopped green or red bell pepper (optional)
sliced black olives (optional)
chopped iceberg lettuce (optional)

1. Coat the slow cooker crock with cooking spray; set aside.
2. In a large mixing bowl, combine all ingredients. Gently press the beef mixture into the slow cooker crock, forming a loaf or a rounded mound shape.
3. Cover and cook on LOW for 8 hours. Let loaf sit, uncovered, for 5 minutes before serving. Serve with your favorite garnishes.

approximate nutritional content
▶ Calories: 427, Protein: 44g, Net Carbs: 6.5g, Fat: 24g, Cholesterol: 248mg, Sodium: 576mg

▶ **serving suggestion**
Use the leftovers from this recipe as a filling in low-carb tortillas, or crumble and use as a salad topper.

american chop suey

▶ **ESTIMATED PREPARATION TIME:** 5 minutes ▶ **COOK TIME:** 8 hours ▶ **SERVINGS:** 6

A perennial favorite, especially among children, this easy dish will be a popular weeknight dinner. Because of the pasta, this dish does not freeze well; eat leftovers for lunch the next day.

1½ cups low-carb elbow macaroni (uncooked)

2 medium onions, finely chopped

1 14.5-ounce can diced tomatoes

1 6-ounce can tomato paste

1 teaspoon black pepper

½ teaspoon kosher salt

¼ teaspoon chili powder

3 teaspoons oregano

bay leaf

¼ teaspoon Tabasco (about 2 shakes)

2 pounds lean ground beef (90% lean), cooked thoroughly

1. Cook the macaroni according to package directions; refrigerate until just before serving.
2. Add all ingredients, except the macaroni, to the slow cooker crock and mix well, breaking up the beef as you stir.
3. Cover and cook on LOW for 8 hours. Stir in cooked macaroni and let mixture sit a few minutes in the slow cooker before serving, to warm the macaroni. Remove bay leaf before serving.

approximate nutritional content
▶ Calories: 464, Protein: 52g, Net Carbs: 12g, Fat: 22g, Cholesterol: 142mg, Sodium: 477mg

▶ **serving suggestion**
American Chop Suey pairs perfectly our Summer Squash Sauté (page 199) or a green salad.

stuffed bell peppers

▶ **ESTIMATED PREPARATION TIME:** 15 minutes ▶ **COOK TIME:** 8 hours ▶ **SERVINGS:** 5

This is a nice dish to put together in the evening, then pop into the slow cooker on your way to work the next day. To do so, prepare the recipe through Step 2, then refrigerate the meat mixture until the morning, when you assemble the dish.

cooking spray
1 pound lean ground beef (90% lean)
½ teaspoon black pepper
1 cube beef bouillon
½ teaspoon Worcestershire sauce
1 14.5-ounce can "petite" diced tomatoes
1 packet dry vegetable soup mix
1 tablespoon minced garlic
¼ cup water
1½ cups shredded Monterey Jack cheese, divided
5 bell peppers (red, green, yellow, or orange)

1. Coat the slow cooker crock with cooking spray; set aside.
2. Spray a large skillet with cooking spray, warm over medium heat and add ground beef, garlic, pepper, and bouillon. Add Worcestershire sauce, tomatoes, dry soup mix, garlic and water; stir well and bring to a simmer. Remove from heat and let mixture cool 10 minutes. Stir in 1 cup of the cheese.
3. Cut the tops off the peppers and pull out the seeds and membranes. Fill pepper cavities with the meat and cheese mixture; sprinkle remaining ½ cup cheese over tops. Place filled peppers in the slow cooker crock.
4. Cover and cook on LOW for 8 hours. Let peppers sit, uncovered, for 10 minutes before serving.

approximate nutritional content
  ▶ Calories: 395, Protein: 31g, Net Carbs: 11g, Fat: 24g, Cholesterol: 104mg, Sodium: 1,145mg

EASY SUBSTITUTION
If you like, use ground turkey (or ground chicken) in place of the ground beef. Doing so will change the approximate nutritional content to:
  ▶ Calories: 362, Protein: 31g, Net Carbs: 11g, Fat: 21g, Cholesterol: 104mg, Sodium: 1,158mg

beef and veggie pie

▶ **ESTIMATED PREPARATION TIME:** 5 minutes ▶ **COOK TIME:** 6 hours ▶ **SERVINGS:** 6

Easy to put together, this recipe provides your daily requirement of protein and veggies all in one dish.

cooking spray

2 pounds lean ground beef (90% lean)

1 1-pound bag frozen mixed vegetables (such as broccoli, cauliflower, and carrots), thawed and drained

1 tablespoon minced garlic

1 tablespoon dried minced onions

3 eggs, beaten

1 8-ounce can tomato sauce

1 packet dry ranch dressing mix

⅛ teaspoon kosher salt

½ teaspoon black pepper

½ teaspoon Tabasco sauce (about 4 shakes)

3 cups (12 ounces) shredded reduced-fat mild cheddar cheese, divided

1. Coat the inside of the slow cooker crock with cooking spray; set aside.

2. In a large mixing bowl, combine all ingredients except 1 cup of the cheese. Gently press the beef mixture into the slow cooker crock.

3. Cover and cook on LOW for 5¾ hours. Sprinkle with remaining cheese and cook 15 minutes more, or until cheese is melted. Turn off slow cooker and let pie rest uncovered for 10 minutes before serving.

4. To serve, cut pie into wedges with a sharp knife. The first piece can be difficult to remove: Use a fork and spatula to get it out of the crock. (There will be cooking juices left in the slow cooker.)

approximate nutritional content

▶ Calories: 655, Protein: 60g, Net Carbs: 14g, Fat: 36g, Cholesterol: 289mg, Sodium: 1,219mg

▶ **serving suggestion**

Got leftovers? A slice of this pie makes a great sandwich when served on low-carb bread or stuffed into a low-carb tortilla!

cheesy mac

▶ **ESTIMATED PREPARATION TIME:** 5 minutes ▶ **COOK TIME:** 8 hours (plus 15 minutes to finish) ▶ **SERVINGS:** 6

This is like Hamburger Helper customized for low-carb diets. If you've got kids, this will become a staple in your recipe repertoire.

2 pounds lean ground beef (90% lean), cooked thoroughly

2 14.5-ounce cans beef broth

1 10.75-ounce can condensed cheddar cheese soup

1 teaspoon black pepper

2 tablespoons dried minced onions

½ teaspoon kosher salt

1½ cups low-carb elbow macaroni, uncooked

⅓ cup light cream

⅔ cup shredded reduced-fat cheddar cheese

1. Add first six ingredients (beef through salt) to the slow cooker crock; mix well. Cover and cook on LOW for 8 hours.

2. When done cooking, stir well and add macaroni. Cover and heat until macaroni is cooked, about 8 to 10 minutes. Add cream and cheese; stir to blend.

approximate nutritional content

▶ Calories: 560, Protein: 56g, Net Carbs: 9g, Fat: 32g, Cholesterol: 175mg, Sodium: 911mg

▶ **cook's tip**
Browning the beef before slow cooking the dish is essential; otherwise, the finished product is greasy.

▶ **serving suggestion**
Serve this with Green Beans with Butter and Hot Sauce (page 202).

beef entrées **81**

mom's classic pot roast

▶ **ESTIMATED PREPARATION TIME:** 5 minutes   ▶ **COOK TIME:** 8 hours   ▶ **SERVINGS:** 6

This has been my dad's favorite entrée as long as I've been around. I've adapted my mom's recipe for the slow cooker. Be sure to use the shoulder chuck roast: It's the leanest and has the least gristle. —KM

1 bottle low-carb beer

2 packets dry onion soup mix

1 teaspoon black pepper

1 cube beef bouillon

¼ teaspoon Tabasco sauce (about 2 shakes)

1 tablespoon quick-cooking tapioca

3-pound chuck shoulder pot roast

1. Add all ingredients, except for the roast, to the slow cooker crock and mix well. Add the roast and turn it, to coat with the sauce. Cover and cook on LOW for 8 hours.

2. Carefully remove the meat from the slow cooker and let it rest, covered with aluminum foil, on a platter or clean cutting board for 10 minutes. Slice the meat (it will break apart easily). Pass the cooking juices along with the meat as "gravy," if desired.

approximate nutritional content

▶ Calories: 387, Protein: 55g, Net Carbs: 3g, Fat: 14g, Cholesterol: 167mg, Sodium: 467mg

▶ **serving suggestion**

Serve this roast with Cheesy Mock Mashed Potatoes (page 170) and Warm Spinach Salad (page 197) for a great American meal.

herbed top round roast

▶ **ESTIMATED PREPARATION TIME:** 10 minutes ▶ **COOK TIME:** 10 hours (plus 15 minutes to finish) ▶ **SERVINGS:** 6

If there was ever a cut of meat that screamed for slow cooking, this is it. This recipe delivers rich, classic beef roast flavor—without heating your oven for hours. —KM

½ cup red wine

½ cup water

1 tablespoon thyme

1 tablespoon rosemary

1 tablespoon black pepper

1 teaspoon kosher salt

2 tablespoons olive oil

3-pound top round roast

5 cloves garlic, halved

½ medium onion, thinly sliced

2 pieces cooked bacon (not crispy)

1. Pour the red wine and water into the slow cooker crock; set aside.
2. In a small bowl, combine the herbs, pepper, salt, and olive oil; stir to combine. Using clean hands, rub the oil and herb mixture all over the beef roast. Place the roast into the slow cooker crock. Sprinkle the garlic and onions around the roast and lay the bacon strips over the top of the roast.
3. Cover and cook on LOW for 10 hours.
4. Before serving, flip the roast over in the slow cooker, then turn the slow cooker off and let the roast rest in the slow cooker for about 15 minutes. Remove roast to a platter and let it drain for a few minutes.
5. To serve, use a sharp knife to slice the meat against the grain. If you like, dip the roast slices into the cooking juices before serving, or serve the cooking juices alongside the beef.

approximate nutritional content
▶ Calories: 485, Protein: 44g, Net Carbs: 3g, Fat: 30g, Cholesterol: 145mg, Sodium: 158mg

> ▶ **serving suggestion**
> Serve this roast with Cheesy Mock Mashed Potatoes (page 170) and steamed broccoli for a nice Sunday supper.

mexican pot roast

▶ **ESTIMATED PREPARATION TIME:** 5 minutes ▶ **COOK TIME:** 8 hours ▶ **SERVINGS:** 6

This is a twist on the traditional pot roast. Consider it when you get a good deal on a roast, or when you aren't necessarily in the mood for "the usual" pot roast.

1 14.5-ounce can red enchilada sauce
1 medium onion, thinly sliced
1 teaspoon black pepper
¼ teaspoon kosher salt
1 teaspoon garlic
1 tablespoon quick-cooking tapioca
3-pound chuck shoulder pot roast

1. Add all ingredients, except for the roast, to the slow cooker crock and mix well. Add the roast and turn it, to coat with the sauce. Using a wooden spoon, push the onions to the side of the roast. Cover and cook on LOW for 8 hours.

2. Carefully remove the meat from the slow cooker and let it rest, covered with aluminum foil, on a platter or clean cutting board for 10 minutes. Slice the meat (it will break apart easily). Top each portion with some of the sauce and onions.

approximate nutritional content
▶ Calories: 461, Protein: 56g, Net Carbs: 6g, Fat: 22g, Cholesterol: 191mg, Sodium: 221mg

▶ **serving suggestion**
Serve this roast with sliced bell peppers, topped with ranch dressing, and some low-carb tortilla chips on the side.

thai green curry beef

▶ **ESTIMATED PREPARATION TIME:** 15 minutes ▶ **COOK TIME:** 8 hours ▶ **SERVINGS:** 5

My husband says this tastes just like what he orders at the Thai restaurant—that's good enough for me! —KB

1 tablespoon plus 1 teaspoon green curry paste

¼ cup beef broth

1 14-ounce can coconut milk

3 tablespoons bottled Thai fish sauce

2 tablespoons Splenda Granular sweetener

2 pounds round steak, cut into bite-sized pieces

1 medium onion, thinly sliced

⅓ cup carrot "matchsticks" (cut from ½ carrot)

1 7-ounce can sliced mushrooms, drained

½ head fresh cauliflower, core removed, broken into florets (about 2 cups)

¾ pound fresh green beans, trimmed (about 4 cups)

2 tablespoons thinly sliced basil leaves (optional)

1. In the slow cooker crock, combine curry paste, broth, coconut milk, fish sauce, and Splenda; mix well with a whisk. Add beef pieces, onions, carrots, mushrooms, and cauliflower pieces; stir to coat ingredients with the sauce.

2. Place green beans on top of mixture and cook on LOW for 8 hours.

3. Before serving, stir the green beans into the dish, and add sliced basil, if desired.

approximate nutritional content
▶ Calories: 506, Protein: 57g, Net Carbs: 9g, Fat: 25g, Cholesterol: 140mg, Sodium: 1,154mg

▶ **cook's tips**

▪ Use fresh vegetables; frozen ones tend to disintegrate in this recipe.

▪ The green beans do tend to lose some of their color during cooking. If you prefer a bright green bean, you can either put them in the crock halfway through the cooking process, or leave them out entirely, steam them on the stove, and then mix them in right before serving.

▪ Do not use "light" coconut milk, as it will separate during cooking.

▶ **about the ingredients**

Green curry paste and fish sauce are available at some larger grocery stores, in the "ethnic" aisle. We use the Thai Kitchen brand.

steak with zucchini, mushrooms, and grape tomatoes

▶ **ESTIMATED PREPARATION TIME:** 10 minutes ▶ **COOK TIME:** 8 hours ▶ **SERVINGS:** 6

No side dish is necessary to round out this meal: everything is here.

2 tablespoons olive oil

2 7-ounce cans sliced mushrooms, drained

1 teaspoon black pepper

1 teaspoon chili powder

1 teaspoon kosher salt

½ teaspoon rosemary, crumbled between fingers

1 tablespoon dried minced onion

1 tablespoon minced garlic

2 tablespoons red wine

2 pounds round steak, cut into 6 pieces

2 pounds zucchini, cut into ¼-inch slices

1 pint grape tomatoes (about 10 ounces)

sour cream (optional)

chopped fresh parsley (optional)

1. Grease the slow cooker crock with the olive oil (leave excess in the crock). Add all ingredients except beef, zucchini, and tomatoes to the crock and stir to combine well.

2. Add the beef, zucchini, and tomatoes; toss with the seasoning mixture.

3. Cover and cook on LOW for 8 hours. Garnish each portion with a dollop of sour cream and a sprinkling of chopped parsley, if desired.

approximate nutritional content
▶ Calories: 327, Protein: 45g, Net Carbs: 7g, Fat: 12g, Cholesterol: 111mg, Sodium: 295mg

---

▶ **cook's tip**

Do not use raw mushrooms in this recipe; they make the sauce too brown. Plus, canned mushrooms are convenient for slow cooker meals; keep some on hand in your pantry.

"steak bomb" casserole

▶ **ESTIMATED PREPARATION TIME:** 10 minutes ▶ **COOK TIME:** 6 hours ▶ **SERVINGS:** 6

When I lived in Boston, a "Steak Bomb" sandwich was a favorite sub shop treat.
Here, we've re-created those great flavors—minus the bread, of course! —KM

2 pounds round cubed pan steak, cut into
    ½-inch strips
1 green bell pepper, cut into thin strips
1 red bell pepper, cut into thin strips
1 medium onion, thinly sliced
1 7-ounce can sliced mushrooms, drained
¾ teaspoon kosher salt
¾ teaspoon black pepper
¼ pound sandwich pepperoni (about 10
    thin slices), cut into ½-inch strips
8 ounces thinly sliced provolone cheese

1. Add all ingredients, except the provolone, to the slow cooker crock and mix well. Cover and cook on LOW for 6 hours.
2. Before serving, stir well. Ladle into individual bowls, top with some of the provolone, then add a little of the cooking juices to melt the cheese.

approximate nutritional content
▶ Calories: 549, Protein: 59g, Net Carbs: 4g, Fat: 31g, Cholesterol: 169mg, Sodium: 1,301mg

ginger garlic beef over braised napa cabbage

▶ **ESTIMATED PREPARATION TIME:** 10 minutes   ▶ **COOK TIME:** 8 hours (plus marinating time of up to 12 hours)
▶ **SERVINGS:** 4

A complete and tasty meal.

for the marinade:
2 tablespoons minced garlic
2 tablespoons minced ginger
2 tablespoons rice vinegar
1 tablespoon soy sauce
1 tablespoon vegetable oil
2 tablespoons olive oil

for the beef and cabbage:
2 pounds London broil steak
½ medium onion, thinly sliced
1 head Napa cabbage (about 1½ pounds), halved lengthwise and thinly sliced
¼ teaspoon salt
2 tablespoons sake
2 tablespoons sesame oil
Soy Crunch Topping (optional) (see page 181)

1. In a small bowl, stir together all marinade ingredients (it will be very thick). Rub the marinade mixture all over the steak and place the steak in a large zip-top bag. Refrigerate overnight (or up to 12 hours).
2. When meat is done marinating, remove bag from the refrigerator; set aside. Add onion to slow cooker crock, then top with the cabbage. Sprinkle the cabbage with the salt, sake, and sesame oil. Using tongs, place the meat on top.
3. Cover and cook on LOW for 8 hours. When done, remove steak with clean tongs and let rest, covered with foil, on a cutting board for 10 minutes.
4. Stir the cabbage and divide it among individual plates. Slice the steak and place it over the cabbage. Garnish each serving with Soy Crunch Topping, if desired.

approximate nutritional content
▶ Calories: 508, Protein: 49g, Net Carbs: 9g, Fat: 28g, Cholesterol: 114mg, Sodium: 460mg

---

▶ **about the ingredients**
Save a little time by using pre-grated ginger. Look for it in your grocery store's produce section.

---

beef bourguignon

▶ **ESTIMATED PREPARATION TIME:** 15 minutes　▶ **COOK TIME:** 8 hours　▶ **SERVINGS:** 6

The extra time spent cooking the mushrooms and browning the beef is well worth it. Our taste-testers ranked this dish high.

8 pieces cooked bacon, chopped

1½ cups red wine

1½ cups beef broth

1 bay leaf

1½ teaspoons thyme

¼ cup tomato paste

1 teaspoon Dijon mustard

2 tablespoons minced garlic

1 teaspoon black pepper

1 tablespoon quick-cooking tapioca

2 tablespoons olive oil, divided

2 10-ounce packages mushrooms, quartered

1½ teaspoons celery salt

2 pounds beef stew meat, fat trimmed

1 1-pound bag frozen pearl onions, thawed

1. Add first 10 ingredients (bacon through tapioca) to the slow cooker crock; stir well to combine.
2. In a medium skillet, over medium heat, warm 1 tablespoon of the oil; add mushrooms and celery salt to the pan. Increase heat to medium–high and cook mushrooms until they are browned and have given off their liquid (about 5 minutes). Drain mushrooms and add them to the slow cooker crock.
3. Return skillet to the heat, add remaining olive oil and brown the beef in the oil. Add the beef and the onions to the slow cooker crock, then stir all ingredients together well.
4. Cover and cook on LOW for 7 hours. Stir stew well and cook 1 hour more. Remove bay leaf before serving.

approximate nutritional content

▶ Calories: 585, Protein: 43g, Net Carbs: 9g, Fat: 37g, Cholesterol: 140mg, Sodium: 1,431mg

▶ **serving suggestion**

Try serving this with a glass of red wine and a cheese course for dessert—*très Français* and *très* low-carb!

classic beef brisket

▶ **ESTIMATED PREPARATION TIME:** 15 minutes ▶ **COOK TIME:** 8 hours (plus marinating time of 12–24 hours)
▶ **SERVINGS:** 4

My friend, John Wilson, relocated to Texas several years ago; this is a slow

cooker low-carb adaptation of his recipe. —KM

for the marinade:

1 cup low-carb beer

1 teaspoon black pepper

2 teaspoons soy sauce

1 tablespoon minced garlic

1 tablespoon dried minced onion

for the brisket:

2 pounds flat-cut beef brisket, fat trimmed

½ cup low-carb beer

3 tablespoons tomato paste

2 cubes beef bouillon

2 teaspoons minced garlic

1 teaspoon Worcestershire sauce

2 teaspoons cider vinegar

1 tablespoon Splenda Granular sweetener

¼ teaspoon dry mustard

2 tablespoons quick-cooking tapioca

1 medium onion, thinly sliced

1. Combine marinade ingredients in a large zip-top bag; add brisket, shake bag gently, then refrigerate overnight (or up to 24 hours).

2. When ready to cook, add all ingredients, except for brisket and the onion slices, to the slow cooker crock and mix well. Remove the brisket from the bag (discard the marinade) and place it in the slow cooker crock. Flip the brisket, to coat with the sauce mixture, and place the onions alongside and on top of the brisket.

3. Cover and cook on LOW for 8 hours. When done cooking, remove the brisket from the slow cooker and let sit on a cutting board for 10 minutes. Slice the meat against the grain. Stir the remaining sauce in the slow cooker; add the brisket slices back to the sauce and stir to coat.

approximate nutritional content
▶ Calories: 411, Protein: 48g, Net Carbs: 10g, Fat: 18g, Cholesterol: 115mg, Sodium: 856mg

▶ **serving suggestion**
Serve with Faux Potato Salad (page 192) and low-carb beer.

▶ **cook's tip**
Brisket really shrinks up when it's cooked, so don't worry if it's a snug fit when you begin cooking—by the end of the cooking process, the meat will be much smaller! If you'd like to make a larger brisket to serve more people, feel free to double the recipe, but make sure your slow cooker can accommodate the larger raw brisket first.

asian-inspired beef ribs

▶ **ESTIMATED PREPARATION TIME:** 5 minutes   ▶ **COOK TIME:** 8 hours   ▶ **SERVINGS:** 4

When my husband brought these to share at work, everyone demanded the recipe. Being the supportive husband he is, he simply told them they'd have to buy the book. —KM

2 tablespoons soy sauce
2 tablespoons minced fresh ginger
2 tablespoons minced garlic
¼ cup hoisin sauce
1 tablespoon Worcestershire sauce
1 tablespoon Splenda Granular sweetener
2 tablespoons sesame oil
2 tablespoons dried minced onion
1 tablespoon oyster sauce
2 tablespoons sake
¼ teaspoon red pepper flakes
4 pounds beef back ribs

1. Mix all ingredients, except the beef ribs, in the slow cooker crock. Add ribs one at a time and coat each with sauce, stacking them in the crock as you go.
2. Cover and cook on LOW 8 hours. When done cooking, remove ribs from the slow cooker and pour cooking juices into a separate container. Allow the fat to separate (there will be a good amount of fat). Skim the fat off, leaving the seasonings and beef drippings.
3. Add the ribs back to the slow cooker; pour the seasonings/drippings mixture on top and serve.

approximate nutritional content
▶ Calories: 553, Protein: 50g, Net Carbs: 11g, Fat: 32g, Cholesterol: 142mg, Sodium: 1,134mg

> ▶ **serving suggestion**
> These ribs are terrific with Asian Broccoli Slaw (page 196).

> ▶ **cook's tip**
> Be aware that these ribs are very tender when cooked this long, and the meat will fall off the bone easily.

bbq beef short ribs with green chilies

▶ **ESTIMATED PREPARATION TIME:** 10 minutes ▶ **COOK TIME:** 8 hours ▶ **SERVINGS:** 4

These are fall-off-the-bone tender. Be sure to have plenty of napkins on hand!

cooking spray
¼ cup tomato paste
2 tablespoons red wine vinegar
1 tablespoon Worcestershire sauce
2 tablespoons soy sauce
2 tablespoons brown mustard
2 tablespoons dried minced onion
2 tablespoons garlic powder
2 teaspoons chili powder
2 teaspoons black pepper
3 tablespoons Splenda Granular sweetener
1 4-ounce can chopped green chilies, drained
4 pounds beef short ribs

1. Coat the slow cooker crock with cooking spray; set aside.
2. In a large mixing bowl, combine all ingredients, except for the ribs; mix well. Using clean hands, spread the mixture over the ribs, coating well. Place the ribs in the slow cooker crock.
3. Cover and cook on LOW for 8 hours. Let the ribs rest, covered, for 5 to 10 minutes before serving. Use tongs to transfer the ribs to a serving platter. Discard the cooking juices, or drain the fat off and serve the skimmed meat juices alongside the ribs for dipping.

approximate nutritional content
▶ Calories: 568, Protein: 56g, Net Carbs: 11g, Fat: 32g, Cholesterol: 158mg, Sodium: 1,006mg

> ▶ **serving suggestion**
> Serve with Creamy Coleslaw (page 195) and some low-carb beer for a great meal!

poultry entrées

chicken with mushrooms and leeks

▶ **ESTIMATED PREPARATION TIME:** 15 minutes ▶ **COOK TIME:** 6 hours ▶ **SERVINGS:** 4

This amazing dish is inspired by the home cooks in Normandy, France. It's enriched and thickened with easy-to-make homemade crème fraîche.

for the crème fraîche:
⅓ cup sour cream
⅓ cup heavy cream

for the chicken:
1 tablespoon butter
1 10-ounce package mushrooms, sliced
2 leeks, cut in half lengthwise, washed thoroughly, and sliced (making half-moons)
2 tablespoons white wine
1 tablespoon Dijon mustard
1 teaspoon thyme
½ teaspoon celery salt
1 teaspoon black pepper
2 pounds skinless, boneless chicken thighs, fat trimmed

1. In a glass jar (such as a clean mayonnaise jar) mix together the sour cream and heavy cream. When the creams are evenly blended, cover the jar and let sit at room temperature. It will be used just prior to serving; it's okay to let it get warm.

2. Grease the slow cooker crock with the butter (leave excess in the crock). Add all ingredients to the slow cooker, except for the chicken and crème fraîche; stir well.

3. Add the chicken and mix everything together. Cover and cook on LOW for 6 hours. When done cooking, use tongs to transfer the chicken pieces to a plate (cover plate to keep warm). Remove ¼ cup of the cooking juices and discard.

4. Stir the crème fraîche into the leek and mushroom mixture, then return the chicken to the slow cooker and stir gently to coat chicken with the sauce.

approximate nutritional content
▶ Calories: 516, Protein: 46g, Net Carbs: 11g, Fat: 31g, Cholesterol: 193mg, Sodium: 548mg

EASY SUBSTITUTION
You can use 2 pounds of chicken breasts instead of the chicken thighs, if you like. This substitution would change the approximate nutritional content to:
▶ Calories: 484, Protein: 61g, Net Carbs: 11g, Fat: 20g, Cholesterol: 193mg, Sodium: 546mg

▶ **serving suggestion**
Steamed green beans would be a perfect side dish.

italian chicken

▶ **ESTIMATED PREPARATION TIME:** 10 minutes   ▶ **COOK TIME:** 8 hours   ▶ **SERVINGS:** 4

My Sicilian mother-in-law, Jo Mayone, created this dish. I simply adapted it for the slow cooker. —KM

½ medium onion, chopped

½ green bell pepper, chopped

2 tablespoons capers, drained

2 tablespoons olive oil

1 anchovy, finely chopped (or 1 tablespoon anchovy paste)

1 tablespoon minced garlic

3 tablespoons tomato paste

1 14.5-ounce can diced tomatoes, drained

1 small can sliced black olives, drained (2.25 ounces drained weight)

1 7-ounce can sliced mushrooms, drained

¼ teaspoon crushed red pepper (or to taste)

1 teaspoon black pepper

½ teaspoon kosher salt

½ teaspoon oregano

2 tablespoons red wine

2 pounds skinless, boneless chicken thighs, fat trimmed

shaved Parmesan cheese (optional)

1. Add all ingredients, except the chicken, to the slow cooker; mix well. Add the chicken and stir to coat it with the other ingredients.
2. Cover and cook on LOW for 8 hours.
3. To serve, transfer chicken thighs to individual plates using tongs. Stir the sauce and spoon a little onto each serving. Garnish with Parmesan shavings, if desired.

approximate nutritional content

▶ Calories: 489, Protein: 47g, Net Carbs: 8.5g, Fat: 28g, Cholesterol: 162mg, Sodium: 912mg

> ▶ **cook's tip**
> Not sure what to do with the leftover green pepper? Cut it into strips and dip into ranch dressing for a snack, or add it to a salad or low-carb sandwich.

poultry entrées   **95**

chicken with sun-dried tomatoes and artichokes

▶ **ESTIMATED PREPARATION TIME:** 5 minutes   ▶ **COOK TIME:** 8 hours   ▶ **SERVINGS:** 4

This dish delivers sophisticated Italian flavors and is a snap to prepare.

cooking spray

1 9-ounce package artichoke hearts, thawed

⅓ cup sun-dried tomatoes, cut into thin strips with kitchen shears

½ pound (½ bag) frozen cauliflower florets, thawed

1 tablespoon minced garlic

1 tablespoon dried oregano

¼ teaspoon kosher salt

½ teaspoon black pepper

¼ cup white wine

2 tablespoons water

2 teaspoons crushed red pepper (optional, for a very spicy dish!)

2 pounds skinless, boneless chicken thighs, fat trimmed

1. Coat the inside of the slow cooker crock with cooking spray. Add all ingredients except the chicken. Stir to thoroughly combine.
2. Add chicken thighs to the mixture and stir together. Cover and cook on LOW for 8 hours.

approximate nutritional content
   ▶ Calories: 543, Protein: 63g, Net Carbs: 7g, Fat: 25g, Cholesterol: 215mg, Sodium: 360mg

EASY SUBSTITUTION

One 8-ounce package of sliced, fresh mushrooms can be substituted for the cauliflower. For this variation the approximate nutritional content would be:
   ▶ Calories: 546, Protein: 63g, Net Carbs: 8g, Fat: 26g, Cholesterol: 215mg, Sodium: 352mg

---

▶ **cook's tip**

Don't worry if the artichokes and cauliflower aren't fully thawed. In fact, pulling them out of the freezer the night before and leaving them on a plate in the refrigerator is fine. They'll be thawed sufficiently the next morning, when you're ready to assemble the recipe.

---

greek chicken

▶ **ESTIMATED PREPARATION TIME:** 10 minutes　▶ **COOK TIME:** 8 hours　▶ **SERVINGS:** 6

This is the specialty of Kim's friend, Dyan Albano. All the classic Greek flavors, all in one pot!

2 tablespoons extra-virgin olive oil

1 tablespoon white wine

⅓ cup sun-dried tomatoes, chopped (or cut with kitchen shears)

2 teaspoons minced garlic

2 teaspoons onion powder

1 tablespoon oregano

½ teaspoon black pepper

¼ teaspoon kosher salt

2 pounds skinless, boneless chicken thighs, fat trimmed

2 pounds Roma tomatoes, seeded and quartered lengthwise (about 5 cups)

1 16-ounce can small, whole black olives, drained

1 cup crumbled feta cheese

1. Add all ingredients, except the chicken, Roma tomatoes, olives, and feta to the slow cooker crock; stir well to combine.

2. Add chicken thighs, Roma tomatoes, and olives to the mixture and stir together. Cover and cook on LOW for 8 hours.

3. Before serving, transfer chicken pieces to individual plates using tongs. Stir in the feta cheese, then spoon the tomato–feta mixture over each serving of chicken.

approximate nutritional content
▶ Calories: 450, Protein: 40g, Net Carbs: 9.5g, Fat: 27g, Cholesterol: 142mg, Sodium: 661mg

rosemary and garlic chicken thighs

▶ **ESTIMATED PREPARATION TIME:** 10 minutes   ▶ **COOK TIME:** 6 hours   ▶ **SERVINGS:** 4

Rosemary and garlic are meant to be together, and a bit of lemon and olive oil pull the flavors together nicely. Leftover chicken is great on top of salad the next day for lunch.

cooking spray

8 cloves of garlic, thinly sliced

1 tablespoon dried rosemary, crushed between your fingers

3 tablespoons olive oil

1 lemon, pierced 12 times and cut in half

½ teaspoon kosher salt

½ teaspoon black pepper

3 tablespoons white wine

2 tablespoons water

2 pounds skinless, boneless chicken thighs, fat trimmed

1. Coat the slow cooker crock with cooking spray. Add all ingredients, except chicken, to the crock and mix well.
2. Add chicken thighs to the slow cooker and toss to coat them with mixture. Cover and cook on LOW for 6 hours.

approximate nutritional content

▶ Calories: 585, Protein: 59g, Net Carbs: 2.5g, Fat: 35g, Cholesterol: 215mg, Sodium: 262mg

▶ **serving suggestion**

To go totally Italian, serve this dish with Broccoli Rabe with Pine Nuts (page 203).

mexican chicken

▶ **ESTIMATED PREPARATION TIME:** 10 minutes   ▶ **COOK TIME:** 8 hours   ▶ **SERVINGS:** 6

You'll say "olé" when you taste this chicken dish paired with black beans and bell peppers. —KM

2 tablespoons tomato paste
1 teaspoon black pepper
1 teaspoon adobo seasoning
1 cup chicken broth
2 teaspoons minced garlic
½ teaspoon chili powder
⅓ teaspoon chili flakes
½ teaspoon cumin
1 tablespoon olive oil
1 medium onion, chopped
2 green bell peppers, chopped
2 pounds skinless, boneless chicken thighs,
　fat trimmed
1 15.5-ounce can black beans, drained
1 4-ounce can chopped green chilies,
　drained
shredded cheddar cheese (optional)
sour cream (optional)

1. Add first eleven ingredients (tomato paste through bell peppers) to the slow cooker crock and mix well.
2. Add chicken thighs and stir well to coat chicken with seasonings; then add black beans and chilies; do not stir.
3. Cover and cook on LOW for 8 hours. Before serving, stir thoroughly. Serve with cheddar cheese and sour cream, if desired.

approximate nutritional content
▶ Calories: 339, Protein: 34g, Net Carbs: 9g, Fat: 16g, Cholesterol: 109mg, Sodium: 811mg

scallion and peanut chicken

▶ **ESTIMATED PREPARATION TIME:** 10 minutes ▶ **COOK TIME:** 8 hours ▶ **SERVINGS:** 4

Oyster sauce is the secret ingredient in this dish. The combination of scallions, peanuts, and oyster sauce creates a flavorful dish that is sure to please even a fussy eater!

3 bunches scallions (green onions), both white and green parts, cut into 1-inch pieces

1 tablespoon sesame oil

1 tablespoon soy sauce

1 tablespoon sake

1 tablespoon minced garlic

½ teaspoon Tabasco sauce (about 4 shakes)

2 tablespoons quick-cooking tapioca

¼ cup oyster sauce

1 tablespoon Splenda Granular sweetener

2 pounds skinless, boneless chicken thighs, fat trimmed

½ cup cocktail peanuts

1. Add all ingredients, except for the chicken and peanuts, to the slow cooker crock; mix well. Add chicken to the crock and stir to coat with the sauce.
2. Cover and cook on LOW for 4 hours. Stir, sprinkle peanuts on top, then cook 4 hours more.
3. To serve, use tongs to place chicken thighs on individual plates, then ladle sauce over chicken.

approximate nutritional content
▶ Calories: 546, Protein: 52g, Net Carbs: 12g, Fat: 31g, Cholesterol: 162mg, Sodium: 1,167mg

▶ **about the ingredients**
Wondering what oyster sauce really is? The condiment known as oyster sauce is made from salt, various seasonings, and yes, oysters. It's found in the "ethnic" section of most grocery stores. Use it when making stir-fries, or for flavoring other Asian-inspired dishes.

▶ **serving suggestion**
This dish is wonderful served over stir-fried shitake mushroom strips, or over low-carb spaghetti.

thai red curry chicken

▶ **ESTIMATED PREPARATION TIME:** 15 minutes ▶ **COOK TIME:** 8 hours ▶ **SERVINGS:** 5

Thai curry does not taste like Indian curry, but it is spicy. Use more or less curry paste to suit your taste. Red curry paste and fish sauce are available at some larger grocery stores in the "ethnic" aisle.

1 tablespoon plus 1 teaspoon red curry paste

¼ cup chicken broth

1 14-ounce can coconut milk

3 tablespoons fish sauce

2 tablespoon Splenda Granular sweetener

2 pounds skinless, boneless chicken thighs, fat trimmed, cut into bite-sized pieces

1 medium onion, halved and thinly sliced

1 8-ounce can bamboo shoots, drained

½ head fresh cauliflower, core removed and broken into florets (about 2 cups)

¾ pound fresh green beans (about 4 cups)

2 tablespoons thinly sliced fresh basil leaves (optional)

1. In the slow cooker crock, combine the curry paste, broth, coconut milk, fish sauce, and Splenda; mix well with a whisk. Add chicken, onions, bamboo shoots, and cauliflower; stir to coat ingredients with sauce.

2. Place green beans on top of mixture and cook on LOW for 8 hours.

3. Before serving, stir the green beans into the dish, and add sliced basil, if desired.

approximate nutritional content
▶ Calories: 549, Protein: 48g, Net Carbs: 7g, Fat: 35g, Cholesterol: 157mg, Sodium: 1,099mg

EASY SUBSTITUTION

If you prefer, you may use 2 pounds of boneless, skinless chicken breast instead of the chicken thighs. This substitution would alter the approximate nutritional content to:
▶ Calories: 478, Protein: 56g, Net Carbs: 7g, Fat: 23g, Cholesterol: 141mg, Sodium: 1,077mg

---

▶ **cook's tips**

■ Use fresh vegetables; frozen ones tend to disintegrate in this recipe.

■ The green beans do tend to lose some of their color during cooking. If you prefer a bright green bean, you can either put them in the crock halfway through the cooking process, or leave them out entirely, steam them on the stove, and then mix them in right before serving.

■ Do not use "lite" coconut milk; it will separate during cooking.

---

martini chicken

▶ **ESTIMATED PREPARATION TIME:** 5 minutes ▶ **COOK TIME:** 8 hours ▶ **SERVINGS:** 4

If you're a fan of the gin martini, you'll love this dish. It's great for entertaining, too!

2 tablespoons butter

2 pounds skinless, boneless chicken thighs, fat trimmed

½ teaspoon black pepper

½ cup good quality gin

3 tablespoons dry vermouth

¼ teaspoon kosher salt

2 tablespoons chicken broth

2 tablespoons dried minced onions

1 cup small stuffed green olives, drained

1. Grease the inside of the slow cooker crock with the butter (leave excess in the crock). Add all ingredients and mix well. Cover and cook on LOW for 8 hours.

2. When done cooking, remove the chicken from the slow cooker using tongs, place on individual plates, then top with spoonfuls of the olives and cooking juices.

approximate nutritional content
▶ Calories: 514, Protein: 48g, Net Carbs: 2g, Fat: 27g, Cholesterol: 177mg, Sodium: 686mg

▶ **serving suggestion**
Our Summer Squash Sauté (page 199) is a perfect match for this dish.

chicken with quinoa

▶ **ESTIMATED PREPARATION TIME:** 10 minutes ▶ **COOK TIME:** 8 hours ▶ **SERVINGS:** 4

Craving your mom's homemade chicken-and-rice casserole? Try this dish for that old-fashioned flavor without the super-high-carb content of rice.

2 tablespoons butter

2 teaspoons minced garlic

1 cup chicken broth

2 tablespoons white wine

¾ teaspoon black pepper

¾ teaspoon kosher salt

⅓ cup plus 1 tablespoon quinoa, rinsed

½ medium onion, finely chopped

2 celery stalks, finely chopped

2 carrots, peeled and finely chopped

2 pounds skinless, boneless chicken thighs, fat trimmed

1 tablespoon chopped fresh parsley (optional)

1. Add all ingredients except for chicken and parsley to the slow cooker crock and mix well to combine. Place chicken thighs on top of the mixture.

2. Cover and cook on LOW for 8 hours. To serve, transfer chicken thighs to individual bowls using tongs. Mix the quinoa and vegetables well, then spoon into the bowls alongside the chicken. Sprinkle with fresh parsley, if desired.

approximate nutritional content
▶ Calories: 510, Protein: 47g, Net Carbs: 15g, Fat: 26g, Cholesterol: 178mg, Sodium: 583mg

> ▶ **about the ingredients**
> Quinoa (pronounced KEEN-wah) is gaining popularity in the U.S., as people come to recognize that it's easy to cook with and combines well with lots of different foods. Quinoa stands out among grains because of its high protein content, it's also a *complete* protein, meaning it contains all of the essential amino acids our bodies need. Quinoa quadruples in volume as it cooks, so you don't need to add very much to most dishes, making it perfect for low-carb dieters.

chicken with summer vegetables

▶ **ESTIMATED PREPARATION TIME:** 15 minutes ▶ **COOK TIME:** 7 hours ▶ **SERVINGS:** 6

If you've got a garden and need to use up your zucchini and yellow squash, this is your recipe! If possible, choose a locally produced *chèvre* (mild goat cheese) to use for the garnish.

2 tablespoons olive oil

6 cups assorted summer squash (about 3 pounds), cut into ½-inch-thick rounds

1 8-ounce can tomato sauce

2 tablespoons white wine

1 tablespoon minced garlic

½ medium onion, thinly sliced

2 celery stalks, sliced ¼-inch thick on the diagonal

¾ teaspoon kosher salt

¾ teaspoon black pepper

1 teaspoon Italian seasoning

1 teaspoon dried oregano

2 pounds skinless, boneless chicken thighs, fat trimmed

1 4-ounce log of chèvre (optional)

1. Add all ingredients except chicken thighs and chèvre to the slow cooker crock; stir well to combine.
2. Add chicken thighs and stir all ingredients together. Cover and cook on LOW for 7 hours.
3. Before serving, stir well. Garnish each serving with a round of goat cheese, if desired.

approximate nutritional content
▶ Calories: 386, Protein: 38g, Net Carbs: 10g, Fat: 20g, Cholesterol: 126mg, Sodium: 422mg

EASY ADD-IN

This dish lends itself well to mushrooms, so feel free to toss in an 8-ounce package of sliced fresh mushrooms. Doing so will change the approximate nutritional content to:
▶ Calories: 385, Protein: 39g, Net Carbs: 10g, Fat: 20g, Cholesterol: 126mg, Sodium: 424mg

chicken with olives and almonds

▶ **ESTIMATED PREPARATION TIME:** 10 minutes ▶ **COOK TIME:** 8 hours ▶ **SERVINGS:** 5

Mediterranean flavor with enough food for a "planned leftover" lunch the next day.

2 tablespoons olive oil

12 large pimento-stuffed olives, drained

¾ cup whole raw almonds

1 tablespoon minced garlic

1 medium onion, halved and thinly sliced

1 teaspoon black pepper

¾ teaspoon celery salt

1 teaspoon cumin

1 teaspoon chili powder

2 tablespoons tomato paste

2 tablespoons white wine

1¼ cups chicken broth

2 pounds skinless, boneless chicken thighs, fat trimmed

1. Grease the slow cooker crock with olive oil (leave excess in the crock). Add all remaining ingredients except for the chicken. Mix well to ensure that the tomato paste has dissolved in the mixture. Add chicken, then toss gently to coat it with the sauce.

2. Cover and cook on LOW for 8 hours. To serve, transfer chicken pieces to individual plates using tongs. Ladle a portion of olive and almond mixture over each serving.

approximate nutritional content
▶ Calories: 507, Protein: 41g, Net Carbs: 7g, Fat: 34g, Cholesterol: 131mg, Sodium: 949mg

---

▶ **serving suggestion**

To incorporate a vegetable into the meal, consider serving the chicken thighs on top of steamed green beans, and then topping it all with the olive and almond mixture.

chicken cacciatore

▶ **ESTIMATED PREPARATION TIME:** 10 minutes   ▶ **COOK TIME:** 8 hours   ▶ **SERVINGS:** 4

This Italian classic "translates" easily into low-carb. The finished product is very saucy, so serve with low-carb pasta, if you like.

1 tablespoon olive oil
1 tablespoon minced garlic
1 28-ounce can crushed tomatoes
1 7-ounce can sliced mushrooms, drained
1 bay leaf
1 tablespoon dried oregano
¾ teaspoon kosher salt
½ teaspoon black pepper
1 tablespoon red wine
2 pounds skinless, boneless chicken thighs, fat trimmed
1 medium onion, halved and thinly sliced
2 green bell peppers, thinly sliced
¼ cup grated Parmesan cheese (optional)

1. Add all ingredients except chicken thighs, onions, and peppers to the slow cooker crock; stir to combine. Add the chicken thighs, onions, and peppers and toss gently with tomato mixture.
2. Cover and cook on LOW for 8 hours. Remove bay leaf before serving, and garnish with grated Parmesan, if desired.

approximate nutritional content
▶ Calories: 488, Protein: 53g, Net Carbs: 11g, Fat: 24g, Cholesterol: 179mg, Sodium: 715mg

> ▶ **serving suggestion**
> Instead of the low-carb pasta, you can serve the Chicken Cacciatore with buttered low-carb toast to soak up all the delicious juices.

creamy layered chicken casserole

▶ **ESTIMATED PREPARATION TIME:** 20 minutes   ▶ **COOK TIME:** 3 hours   ▶ **SERVINGS:** 8

Creamy and rich, these layers of cheese, vegetables, and chicken will please family and guests alike. The crepes in this recipe act like pasta, but without all the carbs.

1 tablespoon butter

2 teaspoon dried minced onions

1 15-ounce tub part-skim ricotta cheese

1 egg, beaten

1¾ cups shredded part-skim mozzarella, divided

2 16-ounce jars of prepared Alfredo sauce

4 premade, packaged crepes

1 16-ounce bag frozen mixed vegetables (broccoli, cauliflower, carrot), thawed and drained

3 cups cooked chicken, cut into bite-sized pieces

¼ cup grated Parmesan cheese

¼ teaspoon black pepper

1. Grease the slow cooker crock with the butter (leave excess in the crock); set aside. In a medium mixing bowl, combine the minced onions, ricotta, egg, and ½ cup of the mozzarella; stir well.

2. Spread ½ cup of the Alfredo sauce in the bottom of the slow cooker crock; top with 1 crepe. Using a spoon, drop ⅓ of the ricotta mixture onto the crepe. Top with ⅓ of the bag of vegetables, then 1 cup of the chicken, ¼ cup of the mozzarella, and another ½ cup Alfredo sauce.

3. Repeat layering 2 more times, starting with a crepe and ending with the last of the Alfredo sauce. Sprinkle the Parmesan cheese, pepper, and last ½ cup of the mozzarella cheese over all.

4. Cover and cook on LOW for 3 hours. When done cooking, let the casserole sit, uncovered, for 15 minutes before serving.

approximate nutritional content
▶ Calories: 606, Protein: 42g, Net Carbs: 13g, Fat: 42g, Cholesterol: 199mg, Sodium: 982mg

EASY SUBSTITUTION

To make this a vegetarian dish, simply omit the chicken and replace it with 1 bag of frozen vegetables that has been thawed overnight in the refrigerator (you'll be using a total of 2 bags of vegetables). The approximate nutritional content of this version is:
▶ Calories: 520, Protein: 28g, Net Carbs: 14g, Fat: 38g, Cholesterol: 152mg, Sodium: 949mg

chicken marsala

▶ **ESTIMATED PREPARATION TIME:** 10 minutes ▶ **COOK TIME:** 4 hours ▶ **SERVINGS:** 4

This is a classic dish that doesn't take too long to make. Start it after lunch on Sunday and you'll be all set come dinner time!

2 tablespoons olive oil

1 10-ounce package white mushrooms, thinly sliced

½ teaspoon kosher salt

2 tablespoons butter

½ cup marsala wine

2 tablespoons quick-cooking tapioca

2 pounds skinless, boneless chicken breasts, fat trimmed, cut into bite-sized pieces

½ teaspoon black pepper

2 tablespoons chopped fresh chives

¼ cup heavy cream

1. In a medium skillet, over medium heat, warm the oil. Add the mushrooms and salt and sauté until the mushrooms are browned, approximately 5 minutes. Drain off any liquid and set mushrooms aside.

2. Grease the slow cooker crock with the butter (leave excess in the crock). In the crock, stir together the marsala and tapioca. Add the chicken pieces and the pepper, and top with the cooked mushrooms.

3. Cover and cook on LOW for 4 hours, stirring once during cooking. Before serving, mix in chives and heavy cream, stirring to combine.

approximate nutritional content
▶ Calories: 485, Protein: 64g, Net Carbs: 7.5g, Fat: 19g, Cholesterol: 205mg, Sodium: 276mg

---

▶ **serving suggestion**
If you like, garnish each serving with some shredded mozzarella cheese. Serve with a portion of low-carb spaghetti and a green salad.

---

chicken piccata

▶ **ESTIMATED PREPARATION TIME:** 10 minutes ▶ **COOK TIME:** 4 hours ▶ **SERVINGS:** 4

Another easy weekend dinner you can pop into the slow cooker after lunch.

If you like classic lemony piccata, you'll love this!

3 tablespoons butter

½ cup white wine

¼ teaspoon Tabasco sauce (about 2 shakes)

2 tablespoons quick-cooking tapioca

2 pounds skinless, boneless chicken breasts, fat trimmed, cut into bite-sized pieces

1 lemon, pierced 6 times with a paring knife, and cut in half

½ teaspoon kosher salt

½ teaspoon black pepper

2 tablespoons capers, drained

2 teaspoons fresh parsley, finely chopped

1. Grease the slow cooker crock with the butter (leave excess in the crock). In a liquid measuring cup, combine the wine, Tabasco sauce, and tapioca; stir and add to the slow cooker crock.

2. Add the chicken pieces and remaining ingredients, except for the parsley.

3. Cover and cook on LOW for 4 hours. When done cooking, remove lemon halves, stir in parsley, and serve.

approximate nutritional content

▶ Calories: 442, Protein: 62g, Net Carbs: 5g, Fat: 16g, Cholesterol: 192mg, Sodium: 457mg

EASY ADD-IN

If you like mushrooms, you could sauté 1 cup of sliced mushrooms in 1 teaspoon of butter, then add to the dish when you add the chicken. This will change the approximate nutritional content to:

▶ Calories: 455, Protein: 62g, Net Carbs: 6g, Fat: 17g, Cholesterol: 195mg, Sodium: 467mg

▶ **serving suggestion**
Serve with low-carb pasta and a garden salad for a delicious meal full of fresh flavors.

3-c casserole (chicken, cheese, and cauliflower)

▶ **ESTIMATED PREPARATION TIME:** 10 minutes ▶ **COOK TIME:** 8 hours ▶ **SERVINGS:** 5

This is a recipe the whole family will enjoy, plus it's an easy way to get the kids to eat some veggies.

cooking spray

2 pounds skinless, boneless chicken breasts, fat trimmed, cut into bite-sized pieces

1 head cauliflower, cored and cut into bite-sized pieces

1 10¾-ounce can condensed cheddar cheese soup

¼ cup chicken broth

¼ teaspoon kosher salt

1½ teaspoons onion powder

½ teaspoon black pepper

½ teaspoon Tabasco sauce (about 4 shakes)

¼ cup heavy cream

1 cup reduced-fat shredded cheddar cheese

1. Coat the slow cooker crock with cooking spray. Add all ingredients, except the cream and shredded cheddar; mix well.
2. Cover and cook on LOW for 8 hours. Before serving, stir in cream and cheese.

approximate nutritional content
▶ Calories: 472, Protein: 59g, Net Carbs: 7.5g, Fat: 21g, Cholesterol: 177mg, Sodium: 952mg

> ▶ **serving suggestion**
> Top each serving with a Crunchy Topping (page 181) for some texture.

chicken pseudo-saltimbocca

▶ **ESTIMATED PREPARATION TIME:** 15 minutes ▶ **COOK TIME:** 4 hours ▶ **SERVINGS:** 6

Our Chicken Pseudo–Saltimbocca has the flavors of real saltimbocca, minus the pricey veal!

cooking spray

¼ cup sun-dried tomatoes (about ½ ounce), chopped

2 pounds skinless, boneless chicken breasts, trimmed and cut into thirds lengthwise

12 thin slices provolone cheese (about 9 ounces)

½ pound sliced prosciutto or good-quality boiled ham

¼ cup fresh sage leaves

½ teaspoon black pepper

¼ cup heavy cream

¼ cup grated Parmesan cheese

▶ **cook's tip**

Don't know what to do with the leftover heavy cream? Whip it with a little Splenda sweetener and serve it over fresh berries for dessert.

▶ **about the ingredients**

Domestic prosciutto works fine in this dish and is much less expensive than imported prosciutto. Save the imported prosciutto to savor by itself.

1. Coat the slow cooker crock with cooking spray; set aside.

2. Slice the cheese in half crosswise, making two stacks. Then cut each stack in half again, making rectangular pieces.

3. Assemble the roll-ups: On a cutting board or clean counter, lay one prosciutto or ham slice with a short end closest to you. Lay two pieces of cheese atop the prosciutto slice, lined up with the bottom edge of the prosciutto slice. Lay one strip of chicken across the cheese. Roll up, starting at bottom edge (chicken may stick out the ends of the roll-up). Place roll-up in the slow cooker crock and repeat until all prosciutto, cheese, and chicken is used, making layers of roll-ups in the crock as you go. Tuck the sage leaves around and between the roll-ups. Sprinkle roll-ups with pepper.

4. Cover and cook on LOW for 4 hours. When done cooking, use tongs to remove the roll-ups to a platter. Turn slow cooker to high. Stir cream and Parmesan into the juices in the crock; cover and cook about 10 minutes.

5. Return roll-ups to the slow cooker crock to coat them with the sauce, and serve.

approximate nutritional content

▶ Calories: 459, Protein: 59g, Net Carbs: 3g, Fat: 22g, Cholesterol: 166mg, Sodium: 1,124mg

poultry entrées **111**

chicken with chinese black bean sauce

▶ **ESTIMATED PREPARATION TIME:** 15 minutes　▶ **COOK TIME:** 6 hours　▶ **SERVINGS:** 5

Chinese black bean sauce and plenty of garlic give this dish an intense and delicious flavor. Look for the sauce in the "ethnic" section of your supermarket, or at an Asian market.

2 tablespoons sesame oil, divided

2 tablespoons sake

¼ cup water

6 cloves of garlic, halved

1 tablespoon minced ginger

1 tablespoon soy sauce

2 tablespoons Chinese black bean sauce

1 teaspoon Splenda Granular sweetener

¼–½ teaspoon crushed red pepper (optional)

3 pounds assorted bone-in chicken pieces (legs, breasts, thighs), skinned, fat trimmed

1. Add all ingredients to the slow cooker crock, except the chicken; mix well.
2. Add the chicken pieces and toss with the sauce to coat chicken thoroughly. Cover and cook on LOW for 6 hours.

approximate nutritional content
▶ Calories: 655, Protein: 76g, Net Carbs: 3g, Fat: 35g, Cholesterol: 242mg, Sodium: 454mg

---

▶ **serving suggestion**

Pan-fried bean sprouts are a great low-carb substitute for the noodles or rice traditionally served with this dish. Or, serve with your favorite stir-fried vegetables.

---

margarita chicken

▶ **ESTIMATED PREPARATION TIME:** 10 minutes ▶ **COOK TIME:** 8 hours ▶ **SERVINGS:** 4

This south-of-the-border treatment takes full advantage of the well-known combination of lime and tequila.

2 tablespoons vegetable oil

1 tablespoon dried minced onion

¼ cup good-quality tequila

½ teaspoon black pepper

½ teaspoon kosher salt

½ teaspoon ground cumin

⅓ cup bottled recaito

3 tablespoons water

2 pounds assorted bone-in chicken pieces, skin removed, fat trimmed

1 lime, pierced 12 times with a paring knife and cut in half

1. Grease the slow cooker crock with the oil (leave excess in the crock). Add all ingredients except the chicken pieces and the lime to the slow cooker crock and mix well to combine.

2. Add chicken pieces and lime and toss to coat. Cover and cook on LOW for 8 hours.

approximate nutritional content

▶ Calories: 421, Protein: 49g, Net Carbs: 1g, Fat: 20g, Cholesterol: 152mg, Sodium: 333mg

▶ **about the ingredients**

Recaito is a bottled seasoning mixture containing cilantro, green pepper, onion, garlic, olive oil, and seasonings. It's a convenient way to add spice to rice-and-bean dishes, as well as soups and stews. Look for it in the "ethnic" aisle of the grocery store; we used the Goya brand.

▶ **serving suggestion**

Try this chicken with Jen's Broccoli Salad (page 189) for a crunchy side dish.

pork entrées

pork smothered in onions

▶ **ESTIMATED PREPARATION TIME:** 15 minutes   ▶ **COOK TIME:** 10 hours   ▶ **SERVINGS:** 4

You might describe this as "French onion soup meets pork cutlets." If you like carmelized onions, you'll love this recipe.

1 tablespoon butter

2 tablespoons olive oil

4 medium onions, sliced into thin rounds or "rings"

1 teaspoon dried thyme

½ teaspoon kosher salt

½ teaspoon black pepper

¼ cup golden sherry

2 pounds pork cutlets

¼ cup shredded Swiss cheese (or Gruyère or Romano)

1. Grease the inside of the slow cooker crock with the butter (leave excess in the crock); set aside.
2. In a large skillet, over medium heat, warm olive oil; add the onions, thyme, salt, and pepper to the pan and sauté until onions are wilted and lightly browned, about 6 minutes. Turn off the heat and add the sherry to the skillet.
3. Place the pork cutlets into the slow cooker crock; top with the onion mixture. Cover and cook on LOW for 10 hours.
4. To serve, garnish each serving with some of the shredded Swiss cheese.

approximate nutritional content
▶ Calories: 570, Protein: 60g, Net Carbs: 6g, Fat: 31g, Cholesterol: 175mg, Sodium: 225mg

---

▶ **serving suggestion**
Jen's Broccoli Salad (page 189) is a good complement to this dish.

---

pork with roasted red peppers and onions

▶ **ESTIMATED PREPARATION TIME:** 10 minutes ▶ **COOK TIME:** 8 hours ▶ **SERVINGS:** 4

This is an easy, tasty dish that's sure to become a favorite. If you like, substitute pork chops (with or without bones) for the pork cutlets.

1 12-ounce jar roasted red peppers, drained and roughly chopped

2 teaspoons minced garlic

2 medium onions, halved and thinly sliced

$\frac{1}{2}$ cup white wine

2 tablespoons capers, drained

2 tablespoons extra-virgin olive oil

$\frac{1}{4}$ teaspoon kosher salt

$\frac{1}{2}$ teaspoon black pepper

2 pounds pork cutlets

1. Add all ingredients, except pork, to the slow cooker crock. Toss to mix. Top with the pork cutlets and stir to coat pork.
2. Cover and cook on LOW for 8 hours.

approximate nutritional content
▶ Calories: 536, Protein: 58g, Net Carbs: 7g, Fat: 26g, Cholesterol: 161mg, Sodium: 615mg

> ▶ **serving suggestion**
> To add even more flavor and color to this entrée, serve it with Marinated Tomato and Feta Salad (page 188).

pork with roasted red peppers, herbs, and olives

▶ **ESTIMATED PREPARATION TIME:** 10 minutes ▶ **COOK TIME:** 8 hours ▶ **SERVINGS:** 4

A flavorful variation on Pork with Roasted Red Peppers and Onions (page 117).

1 12-ounce jar roasted red peppers, drained and roughly chopped

2 teaspoons minced garlic

2 medium onions, halved and thinly sliced

½ cup white wine

1 8-ounce can whole black olives, drained

2 tablespoons capers, drained

2 tablespoons extra-virgin olive oil

¼ teaspoon kosher salt

½ teaspoon black pepper

1 teaspoon dried rosemary

1½ teaspoons thyme

2 pounds pork cutlets

1. Add all ingredients, except the pork, to the slow cooker crock. Toss to mix. Top with the pork cutlets and stir.
2. Cover and cook on LOW for 8 hours.

approximate nutritional content
▶ Calories: 587, Protein: 59g, Net Carbs: 8g, Fat: 31g, Cholesterol: 161mg, Sodium: 986mg

▶ **serving suggestion**
This recipe is great when served with low-carb tortillas that have been brushed with olive oil and heated in a hot frying pan.

pork cutlets with apples and mustard

▶ **ESTIMATED PREPARATION TIME:** 10 minutes　▶ **COOK TIME:** 8 hours　▶ **SERVINGS:** 4

A great fall dinner; spicy mustard and sweet apples are a perfect pair.

2 tablespoons butter

2 tablespoons white wine

2 tablespoons apple cider

2 tablespoons quick-cooking tapioca

2 tablespoons Dijon mustard

½ teaspoon black pepper

¼ teaspoon kosher salt

2 pounds pork cutlets

1 medium apple, cored and thinly sliced (leave skin on)

½ medium onion, thinly sliced

1. Grease the inside of the slow cooker crock with the butter (leave excess in the crock). Add all ingredients to the slow cooker crock, except the pork, apple, and onions; mix well.

2. Add pork, onions, and apples, and toss gently to combine. Cover and cook on LOW for 8 hours.

3. To serve, divide pork among plates, then stir the sauce well to blend it before spooning it over the cutlets.

approximate nutritional content
▶ Calories: 595, Protein: 67g, Net Carbs: 12g, Fat: 29g, Cholesterol: 210mg, Sodium: 413mg

---

▶ **serving suggestion**
Green Beans with Bacon (page 201) or some sauerkraut go nicely with this dish.

---

pork cutlets with brussels sprouts, almonds, and bacon

▶ **ESTIMATED PREPARATION TIME:** 10 minutes ▶ **COOK TIME:** 8 hours ▶ **SERVINGS:** 5

"Mmmmm!" was the consensus among our recipe testers. The Dijon sauce coats the pork and seasons the sprouts.

2 tablespoons butter

1 tablespoon Dijon mustard

3 tablespoons mayonnaise

3 tablespoons white wine

½ teaspoon onion powder

½ teaspoon black pepper

½ teaspoon kosher salt

¼ teaspoon Tabasco sauce (about 2 shakes)

2 tablespoons water

2 pounds pork cutlets

2 10-ounce packages frozen brussels sprouts

¼ cup bacon pieces (or 2 slices cooked bacon, chopped)

¼ cup sliced almonds

1. Grease the slow cooker crock with the butter (leave excess in the crock). Add all ingredients to the slow cooker crock, except the pork, brussels sprouts, bacon, and almonds; blend mixture using a whisk.

2. Lay pork over the Dijon mixture, then top with brussels sprouts and sprinkle with bacon and almonds.

3. Cover and cook on LOW for 8 hours. To serve, spoon brussels sprouts onto plates, then remove pork cutlets with tongs and place alongside the sprouts on each plate.

4. Whisk the sauce remaining in the slow cooker crock; it will come together easily. Spoon a little sauce over each serving of pork and sprouts.

approximate nutritional content
▶ Calories: 533, Protein: 52g, Net Carbs: 5g, Fat: 31g, Cholesterol: 148mg, Sodium: 379mg

▶ **cook's tips**
■ Look for real bacon pieces in the salad dressing aisle.
■ Frozen brussels sprouts are preferable in this recipe, as they hold together well and are convenient.

orange pork

▶ **ESTIMATED PREPARATION TIME:** 5 minutes   ▶ **COOK TIME:** 8 hours   ▶ **SERVINGS:** 4

This kid-friendly dish is easily adaptable to chicken; just substitute an equal amount of boneless chicken breast for the pork.

2 tablespoons butter

½ teaspoon kosher salt

½ teaspoon black pepper

1 teaspoon dried minced onions

2 teaspoons minced garlic

2 tablespoons white wine

2 tablespoons orange juice

¼ teaspoon chili powder

¼ teaspoon Tabasco sauce (about 2 shakes)

2 pounds boneless center-cut pork chops

1 navel orange, pierced 12 times and cut in half

2 tablespoons chopped fresh chives (optiona)

1. Grease the slow cooker crock with the butter (leave excess in the crock). Add all remaining ingredients, except the orange and the pork chops, to the crock and stir to combine.

2. Add the chops and stir to coat with the seasoning mixture. Push orange pieces down into the seasoned chops.

3. Cover and cook on LOW for 8 hours. When done cooking, garnish with chopped chives, if desired.

approximate nutritional content
   ▶ Calories: 588, Protein: 55g, Net Carbs: 6g, Fat: 36g, Cholesterol: 160mg, Sodium: 214mg

EASY SUBSTITUTION
During tangerine season (winter months, for most people), feel free to use a tangerine in place of the navel orange.

▶ **serving suggestion**
Super Delish Snap Peas (page 198) or Tomato, Basil, and Mozzarella Salad (page 191) are wonderful with this flavorful entrée.

pork with scallions and shitake mushrooms

▶ **ESTIMATED PREPARATION TIME:** 15 minutes   ▶ **COOK TIME:** 8 hours   ▶ **SERVINGS:** 5

This distinctive dish is great on its own, and even better over low-carb pasta.

1 tablespoon soy sauce

1 tablespoon grated fresh ginger

1 tablespoon minced garlic

2 tablespoons sake

¼ cup hoisin sauce

1 tablespoons sesame oil

1 tablespoon vegetable oil

¼ teaspoon crushed red pepper flakes

2 pounds boneless, center-cut pork chops, cut into thin strips

½ pound shitake mushrooms, stems removed, caps thinly sliced

2 bunches of scallions, both green and white parts, cut into 1-inch pieces

1. Add first eight ingredients (soy sauce through red pepper) to the slow cooker crock and mix well. Add pork, mushrooms, and scallions; stir gently to coat with the sauce.

2. Cover and cook on LOW for 8 hours. Stir well before serving.

approximate nutritional content
▶ Calories: 486, Protein: 56g, Net Carbs: 13g, Fat: 21g, Cholesterol: 154mg, Sodium: 525mg

smoked pork chops in sauerkraut

▶ **ESTIMATED PREPARATION TIME:** 10 minutes   ▶ **COOK TIME:** 8 hours   ▶ **SERVINGS:** 6

This Alsatian-inspired dish is easy and delicious for a weeknight dinner. Look for fresh sauerkraut near the refrigerated pickles.

1 tablespoon butter

1 medium onion, halved and chopped

2 pounds fresh sauerkraut (rinsed in a colander to reduce sodium content, if desired)

2 tablespoons white wine

½ teaspoon kosher salt

¼ teaspoon garlic powder

½ teaspoon black pepper

2 pounds smoked pork chops

1. Grease the slow cooker crock with the butter (leave excess in the crock). Add all remaining ingredients, except chops, to the crock and stir to combine.
2. Push chops down into the sauerkraut mixture. Cover and cook on low for 8 hours.

approximate nutritional content
▶ Calories: 481, Protein: 32g, Net Carbs: 3g, Fat: 35g, Cholesterol: 93mg, Sodium: 2,759mg

---

▶ **serving suggestion**

A dollop of sour cream is a nice garnish for this dish and also tones down the spiciness and acidity of the sauerkraut. Kids may especially like this addition.

---

pork with prosciutto and artichoke hearts

▶ **ESTIMATED PREPARATION TIME:** 10 minutes ▶ **COOK TIME:** 8 hours ▶ **SERVINGS:** 5

This dish features plenty of bold Italian flavors that are sure to please.

1 14-ounce can artichoke hearts, drained and quartered

2 tablespoons olive oil

½ medium onion, thinly sliced

½ teaspoon black pepper

1 teaspoon garlic powder

½ teaspoon red pepper flakes

1 teaspoon oregano

2 tablespoons white wine

4 ounces prosciutto, chopped

2 pounds boneless center-cut pork chops, fat trimmed

¼ cup heavy cream

¼ cup grated Romano cheese

1. Add all ingredients, except for cream and cheese, to the slow cooker crock; mix well. Make sure chops are lying flat in the crock.
2. Cover and cook on LOW for 8 hours.
3. When done cooking, use tongs to transfer pork chops to a platter. Add the cream and Romano cheese to the crock; stir well to combine them with the cooking juices. Return pork chops to the crock to coat with the sauce.

approximate nutritional content
▶ Calories: 498, Protein: 56g, Net Carbs: 6g, Fat: 25g, Cholesterol: 162mg, Sodium: 684mg

EASY SUBSTITUTION

Boneless, skinless chicken thighs (fat trimmed) can be substituted for the pork chops, if desired. Doing so will change the approximate nutritional content to:
▶ Calories: 443, Protein: 42g, Net Carbs: 6g, Fat: 26g, Cholesterol: 155mg, Sodium: 691mg

EASY ADD-IN

If you like, add a 14.5-ounce can of diced tomatoes (drained) to the mixture. Doing so will change the approximate nutritional content to:
▶ Calories: 512, Protein: 57g, Net Carbs: 9g, Fat: 25g, Cholesterol: 162mg, Sodium: 804mg

pork chops with pecans and chilies

▶ **ESTIMATED PREPARATION TIME:** 5 minutes ▶ **COOK TIME:** 8 hours ▶ **SERVINGS:** 6

This is an intense dish in which the chilies, spices, and pecans create layers of flavors and texture.

cooking spray

2 4-ounce cans chopped green chilies

⅛ teaspoon cinnamon

½ teaspoon black pepper

½ teaspoon kosher salt

1½ teaspoons chili powder

½ cup low-carb beer

2 tablespoons minced garlic

2 teaspoons dried, minced onions

2 tablespoons tomato paste

2 pounds boneless center-cut pork chops, fat trimmed

1 cup pecans

½ cup water

1. Coat the slow cooker crock with cooking spray. Add next nine ingredients (chilies through tomato paste) to the crock and mix well.

2. Add the pork and toss to coat well with seasoning mixture. Sprinkle pecans over the pork.

3. Cover and cook on LOW for 8 hours. When done cooking, use tongs to transfer pork to a serving platter. Stir in the water to thin out the sauce, and spoon sauce over chops.

approximate nutritional content
▶ Calories: 479, Protein: 38g, Net Carbs: 5g, Fat: 33g, Cholesterol: 96mg, Sodium: 255mg

> ▶ **serving suggestion**
> A "cool" side dish, such as Kim's Mom's Cucumber Salad (page 193) is especially refreshing with this dish.

classic country-style bbq pork ribs

▶ **ESTIMATED PREPARATION TIME:** 10 minutes ▶ **COOK TIME:** 8 hours ▶ **SERVINGS:** 4

This recipe is one of my husband's favorites; it can easily be doubled if you have company coming, too. Be aware that, unlike grilled or smoked ribs, the meat on these ribs falls off the bone when properly cooked. Don't worry, that's supposed to happen! —KM

cooking spray

1 tablespoon garlic powder

1 teaspoon paprika

2 tablespoons Splenda Granular sweetener

1 tablespoon chili powder

1 tablespoon black pepper

½ teaspoon kosher salt

½ teaspoon cayenne pepper

½ teaspoon cumin

2 tablespoons low-carb beer

2 tablespoons brown mustard

1 tablespoon Worcestershire sauce

1 medium onion, thinly sliced

2 pounds country-style pork spareribs

1. Coat the slow cooker crock with cooking spray; set aside.

2. In a small mixing bowl, combine all remaining ingredients except onions and ribs; blend well to make a paste. Using clean hands, rub spice mixture all over ribs, one at a time, then place into slow cooker. Continue with all the ribs and remaining spice mixture. Sprinkle onions on top of ribs in slow cooker.

3. Cover and cook on LOW heat for 8 hours. To serve, remove ribs to a platter (they are super-tender; the meat will fall off the bone), skim the fat from the drippings, and pass the drippings separately as an extra BBQ sauce, if desired.

approximate nutritional content

▶ Calories: 407, Protein: 42g, Net Carbs: 5.5g, Fat: 22g, Cholesterol: 134mg, Sodium: 411mg

▶ **serving suggestion**

These spicy ribs go nicely with Zippy Coleslaw (page 194) and a low-carb beer.

rum and molasses baby back ribs

▶ **ESTIMATED PREPARATION TIME:** 15 minutes ▶ **COOK TIME:** 8 hours ▶ **SERVINGS:** 4

The spiced rum and other sweet spices in this recipe combine really well with the pork, making a delish sauce. —KM

2 tablespoons molasses

¼ cup spiced rum

1 tablespoon dried minced onions

1 tablespoon minced garlic

1 tablespoon black pepper

2 tablespoons Splenda Granular sweetener

pinch cinnamon

1 teaspoon paprika

1 teaspoon chili powder

1 tablespoon soy sauce

1 tablespoon cider vinegar

2 tablespoons tomato paste

4 pounds baby back pork ribs, cut into sections of 3 to 4 bones each

1. Add all ingredients, except for pork ribs, to the slow cooker crock; mix well. Add the rib sections, one at a time, flipping them over to coat with the sauce.

2. Cover and cook on LOW for 8 hours. Skim off fat and use the remaining drippings as a dipping sauce, if desired.

approximate nutritional content
▶ Calories: 611, Protein: 60g, Net Carbs: 11g, Fat: 31g, Cholesterol: 194mg, Sodium: 476mg

---

▶ **cook's tips**

■ Our butcher says that 1 pound of baby back ribs per person is enough, but that "hungry big guys" may want more than that. This recipe can easily be doubled to accommodate those "hungry guys,"—just make sure your slow cooker can hold that much food!

■ This recipe is most easily done by hand (dragging the ribs through the sauce). Wash your hands first, then don't fret about getting your hands dirty. If you'd rather not use your hands, a pastry brush works well.

▶ **serving suggestions**

Creamy Coleslaw (page 195) or Faux Potato Salad (page 192) are both good choices with these ribs.

chili-rubbed shredded pork

▶ **ESTIMATED PREPARATION TIME:** 10 minutes ▶ **COOK TIME:** 8 hours ▶ **SERVINGS:** 6

This is so easy and versatile, it's sure to become a favorite.

1 4-ounce can chopped green chilies

2 teaspoons chili powder

2 teaspoons garlic powder

1 teaspoon soy sauce

1 teaspoon black pepper

2 teaspoons onion powder

1 teaspoon adobo seasoning

2 teaspoons oregano

1 tablespoon vegetable oil

1 teaspoon cumin

3-pound boneless prime rib pork oven roast

1. In a small mixing bowl, combine all ingredients except for the pork roast. Using clean hands, rub the mixture all over the pork, then place the roast in the slow cooker crock.

2. Cover and cook on LOW for 8 hours. Let the roast rest, covered, for 10 minutes.

3. Lift the roast out of the slow cooker and transfer it to a cutting board. Shred the pork, using two forks. Add the shredded pork back to the slow cooker to absorb some of the cooking juices. Transfer to individual bowls, to serve.

approximate nutritional content

▶ Calories: 334, Protein: 47g, Net Carbs: 3g, Fat: 14g, Cholesterol: 118mg, Sodium: 385mg

▶ **serving suggestions**

■ Serve shredded pork with low-carb tortillas, cheese, chopped avocado, chopped tomato, and lettuce.

■ Use the pork as a sandwich stuffer, either hot or cold.

■ Top a salad with the shredded pork.

seafood entrées

swordfish with pesto

▶ **PREPARATION TIME:** 5 minutes ▶ **COOKING TIME:** 4 hours ▶ **SERVINGS:** 4

Fish in the slow cooker? As far as we know, celebrated cookbook author Lora Brody was the first to do it, in her book *Slow Cooker Cooking* (2001). As you know, fish is a great source of lean protein, as well as healthy omega-3 fatty acids.

⅓ cup pesto (homemade or purchased), divided

2 pounds swordfish steaks, patted dry with a paper towel

1. Spread 3 tablespoons of the pesto over one side of the fish steaks. Place the fish, pesto–side up, in the slow cooker crock.
2. Cover and cook on LOW for 4 hours.
3. Before serving, dab remaining pesto over the fish.

approximate nutritional content
▶ Calories: 397, Protein: 53g, Net Carbs: 1g, Fat: 19g, Cholesterol: 103mg, Sodium: 330mg

▶ **serving suggestion**
This dish is a perfect match for Warm Asparagus and Red Pepper Salad (page 190).

sesame tuna with bok choy and shitake mushrooms

▶ **PREPARATION TIME:** 15 minutes (plus marinating time of up to 1 hour)   ▶ **COOKING TIME:** 4 hours   ▶ **SERVINGS:** 4

This Asian-influenced dish is just as delicious with salmon fillets as it is with tuna.

for marinade:

1 tablespoon minced fresh ginger

1 tablespoon minced garlic

3 tablespoons sake

3 tablespoons soy sauce

¼ cup toasted sesame oil

2 tablespoons rice vinegar

1 teaspoon onion powder

1 teaspoon Splenda Granular sweetener

for the fish:

2 pounds tuna steaks (or salmon fillets, skinned)

¾ pound fresh shitake mushrooms, stems removed, thinly sliced

1 head bok choy, washed and thinly sliced (separate green parts from white parts)

2 tablespoons toasted sesame seeds (optional)

1. Mix together all of the marinade ingredients and pour into a zip-top, gallon-sized food storage bag (or pour into a glass dish). Add tuna and swish around to make sure the fish is coated with marinade. Let fish sit out in the bag while you prepare the rest of the recipe, or place bag in the refrigerator and let marinate for up to 1 hour.

2. Place the shitake mushrooms into the slow cooker crock. Top with the white bok choy pieces, then the leafy green bok choy pieces, and then place the fish over the vegetables. Pour the marinade over all.

3. Cover and cook on LOW for 4 hours. To serve, fill individual bowls with bok choy and mushrooms, then top with fish and sprinkle with toasted sesame seeds, if desired.

approximate nutritional content

▶ Calories: 574, Protein: 3g, Net Carbs: 17g, Fat: 27g, Cholesterol: 98mg, Sodium: 922mg

citrus salmon

▶ **PREPARATION TIME:** 15 minutes ▶ **COOKING TIME:** 4 hours (plus marinating time of at least 6 hours) ▶ **SERVINGS:** 4

This is a zesty, tasty way to prepare salmon. Leftovers (if there are any) are perfect as a topping for salad.

for the marinade:

1 tablespoon honey

juice of ½ lemon

juice of ½ lime

juice of ½ orange

1 teaspoon minced garlic

2 teaspoons soy sauce

1 tablespoon vegetable oil (do not use olive oil)

¼ teaspoon Tabasco sauce (about 2 shakes)

¼ teaspoon black pepper

for the fish:

2 pounds salmon fillets, skinned

½ lemon, sliced

½ lime, sliced

½ orange, sliced

1. In a large zip-top bag, combine marinade ingredients; place salmon into the bag and refrigerate for at least 6 hours (preferably overnight).
2. When done marinating, remove salmon from bag and place in slow cooker crock (discard marinade). Place slices of lemon, lime, and orange around the fish in the crock.
3. Cover and cook on LOW for 4 hours. When done, let fish sit, uncovered, for 10 minutes before serving.

approximate nutritional content

▶ Calories: 420, Protein: 51g, Net Carbs: 8g, Fat: 20g, Cholesterol: 140mg, Sodium: 285mg

---

▶ **cook's tips**

◼ Getting the skin off the salmon fillet can be difficult. Most places will skin the fillets for you after they weigh your fish—take advantage of this service.

◼ Use a mild-flavored vegetable oil in this recipe; olive oil will overpower the delicate citrus flavors.

▶ **serving suggestion**

Serve with blanched broccoli that's topped with our Sesame-Soy Dressing (page 185).

---

miso-rubbed salmon

▶ **PREPARATION TIME:** 5 minutes (plus marinating time of at least 4 hours)   ▶ **COOKING TIME:** 4 hours   ▶ **SERVINGS:** 4

Miso is a cultured soybean-and-rice paste that adds a definite yet delicate flavor to the salmon.

1 tablespoon soy sauce

1 tablespoon sake

1 tablespoon miso (yellow or red)

1 tablespoon sesame oil

1 teaspoon minced fresh ginger

2 pounds salmon fillets, skin removed

1 scallion, sliced (optional)

1. In a small bowl, stir the soy sauce, sake, miso, sesame oil, and ginger into a paste. Using clean hands, rub the paste onto the salmon, then place the salmon on a plate (cover with plastic wrap) or in a large zip-top plastic bag; refrigerate at least 4 hours and not longer than overnight.
2. When fish is done marinating, transfer salmon to the slow cooker crock (discard marinade). Cover and cook on LOW for 4 hours.
3. Before serving, sprinkle sliced scallions over the salmon, if desired.

approximate nutritional content
▶ Calories: 405, Protein: 51g, Net Carbs: 1.5g, Fat: 20g, Cholesterol: 140mg, Sodium: 526mg

▶ **serving suggestion**
Asian Broccoli Slaw (page 196) is an appropriate way to round out this meal.

food for entertaining

buttered roasted almonds

▶ **ESTIMATED PREPARATION TIME:** 10 minutes ▶ **COOK TIME:** 2 hours ▶ **SERVINGS:** 12

These are the absolute best—easy and so delicious. They'll be a staple item in your house once you taste them! —KB

3 tablespoons butter
1 pound whole, raw almonds (or pecans, if you prefer)
1½ tablespoons kosher salt

1. Turn slow cooker to HIGH and place butter in crock; allow butter to melt. Once melted, turn slow cooker to LOW. Add the nuts and stir to coat with the butter.
2. Cover and cook on LOW for 2 hours, stirring several times during cooking.
3. When done cooking, add the salt and toss the nuts well to coat with salt. Let nuts cool, uncovered, then store in a tightly sealed container until serving.

approximate nutritional content
▶ Calories: 248, Protein: 8g, Net Carbs: 4g, Fat: 23g, Cholesterol: 8mg, Sodium: 213mg

▶ **cook's tip**
This recipe can easily be doubled if you have a large crowd coming over (or if you just want to have them on hand for snacking at home!).

almonds diablo

▶ **ESTIMATED PREPARATION TIME:** 5 minutes ▶ **COOK TIME:** 2 hours ▶ **SERVINGS:** 16

Spicy, nutty perfection! These nuts don't seem spicy right off, but they catch up to you. If you want to live dangerously, increase the cayenne a tad, and have a cold drink handy.

20 ounces (about 4 cups) whole raw
   almonds
¼ cup (½ stick) butter, melted
1½ teaspoons cayenne pepper
1 tablespoon Tabasco sauce

1. Add nuts to the slow cooker crock.
2. In a small bowl, combine the remaining ingredients and mix well. Pour the mixture over the almonds and stir to coat the nuts thoroughly.
3. Cover and cook on LOW for 2 hours. Stir several times during cooking.

approximate nutritional content
   ▶ Calories: 235, Protein: 7g, Net Carbs: 4g, Fat: 21g, Cholesterol: 8mg, Sodium: 39mg

EASY SUBSTITUTION
You can easily replace some or all of the almonds with raw peanuts or cashews for a spicy, crowd-pleasing mixed-nut treat.

▶ **cook's tip**
These are great as a snack by themselves; they also are a flavorful addition to salad.

cinnamon walnuts

▶ **ESTIMATED PREPARATION TIME:** 10 minutes ▶ **COOK TIME:** 2½ hours ▶ **SERVINGS:** 12

My mother likes these so much, she has a standing order. —KM

1 pound raw walnut halves

¼ cup (½ stick) butter, melted

2 teaspoons cinnamon, divided

1 teaspoon sugar, divided

1 tablespoon Splenda Granular sweetener

1 teaspoon vanilla

1. Place the walnuts in the slow cooker crock.
2. In a small bowl, mix together the butter, 1 teaspoon cinnamon, ½ teaspoon sugar, Splenda, and vanilla. Mix well and pour over the walnuts in the slow cooker, stirring well to coat the nuts.
3. Cover and cook on LOW for 2½ hours. When done cooking, sprinkle the remaining sugar and cinnamon over the nuts, toss well, and serve warm, or allow to cool, uncovered, until serving time.

approximate nutritional content
▶ Calories: 267, Protein: 9g, Net Carbs: 3g, Fat: 25g, Cholesterol: 10mg, Sodium: 40mg

▶ **cook's tip**

Don't worry about the small amount of real sugar in this recipe; it makes the cinnamon coat the nuts so much better than without it. The carbs are still low, so relax!

▶ **serving suggestion**

These nuts are a great snack as is, but they're also delicious sprinkled over cottage cheese or salad.

curried mixed nuts

▶ **ESTIMATED PREPARATION TIME:** 10 minutes ▶ **COOK TIME:** $2\frac{1}{2}$ hours ▶ **SERVINGS:** 20

Inspired by a recipe for Spiced Holiday Nuts created by fellow Mainer and accomplished culinary professional Kathy Gunst, these nuts can be downright addictive! For the original recipe by Gunst, see *Bon Appetit* (Nov. 1998) or her book *Relax, Company's Coming!* (2001).

¼ cup canola oil

3 tablespoons butter, melted

1½ teaspoons ground ginger

1½ teaspoons curry powder

1 teaspoon cayenne pepper

1 teaspoon kosher salt

¼ teaspoon Splenda Granular sweetener

10 ounces whole raw almonds

8 ounces raw cashews

8 ounces raw pecan halves

1. In a small bowl, combine oil, butter, spices, and Splenda; mix well.
2. Place nuts in the slow cooker crock; pour butter mixture over nuts and toss well to coat nuts with seasonings.
3. Cover and cook on LOW for 2½ hours, stirring several times during cooking.

approximate nutritional content
▶ Calories: 265, Protein: 6g, Net Carbs: 7g, Fat: 25g, Cholesterol: 5mg, Sodium: 45mg

EASY SUBSTITUTION
If you prefer, substitute raw peanuts for the pecans or cashews.

maple pecans

▶ **ESTIMATED PREPARATION TIME:** 10 minutes   ▶ **COOK TIME:** 2½ hours   ▶ **SERVINGS:** 12

This special recipe demands real maple syrup or it won't succeed. Don't worry, it's worth it!

¼ cup (½ stick) butter
¼ cup real maple syrup
¼ teaspoon vanilla
½ teaspoon maple extract
1 pound raw pecan halves

1. Place the butter in the slow cooker crock and turn it to HIGH until butter melts. Then turn slow cooker to LOW and add maple syrup, vanilla, and maple extract; mix well.
2. Add nuts and toss to coat them with the syrup mixture.
3. Cover and cook on LOW for 2½ hours, stirring several times during cooking.

approximate nutritional content
▶ Calories: 304, Protein: 3g, Net Carbs: 9g, Fat: 29g, Cholesterol: 10mg, Sodium: 40mg

EASY SUBSTITUTION
Don't like pecans? Almonds or walnuts would be a perfect substitute.

▶ **cook's tip**
Do not taste these nuts directly out of the slow cooker—they're too hot! Let them cool first.

glazed sweet and spicy pecans

▶ **ESTIMATED PREPARATION TIME:** 5 minutes ▶ **COOK TIME:** 2 hours ▶ **SERVINGS:** 12

Initially sweet, these pecans pack a spicy finish!

3 tablespoons butter

2 tablespoons vegetable oil

2 tablespoons Splenda Granular sweetener

2 tablespoons honey

¼ teaspoon kosher salt

1¼ teaspoons cayenne pepper

1 teaspoon dry mustard

1 pound raw pecan halves

1. Place the butter in the slow cooker crock and turn it to HIGH until butter melts; turn slow cooker to LOW and add the oil and all remaining ingredients, except for the pecans. Stir well.

2. Add the pecans and stir to coat them well with the spice mixture.

3. Cover and cook on LOW 2 hours, stirring several times during cooking.

approximate nutritional content

▶ Calories: 310, Protein: 3g, Net Carbs: 8g, Fat: 31g, Cholesterol: 8mg, Sodium: 40mg

miso soup with tofu and scallions

▶ **ESTIMATED PREPARATION TIME:** 5 minutes　▶ **COOK TIME:** 4 hours　▶ **SERVINGS:** 6

This is the easiest soup ever, and the resulting flavors are both delicate and delicious. It makes a wonderful first course when entertaining. For an Asian-inspired dinner, prepare this a day ahead, refrigerate it, then warm it up when guests arrive. Follow up with our Sesame Tuna with Bok Choy and Shitake Mushrooms (page 131), to make double use of your slow cooker!

⅓ cup plus 1 tablespoon miso (yellow or red)

9 cups water

½ pound extra-firm tofu, cut into ¼-inch cubes

4 whole scallions, thinly sliced

1. In the crock of the slow cooker, mix together the miso and water. Add the tofu cubes. Cover and cook on LOW for 4 hours.
2. Before serving, stir in the scallion pieces. This soup separates quickly; just stir it again before serving.

approximate nutritional content
▶ Calories: 91, Protein: 8g, Net Carbs: 6g, Fat: 4g, Cholesterol: 0mg, Sodium: 615mg

> ### ▶ about the ingredients
> Can't find miso? It's typically found in the produce section of grocery stores, near other Asian foods and ingredients. Ask an employee if you have trouble finding it.

babaghanoush

▶ **ESTIMATED PREPARATION TIME:** 15 minutes   ▶ **COOK TIME:** 6 hours (plus overnight chilling time)   ▶ **SERVINGS:** 16

This Middle Eastern spread is perfect as a dip for veggies or grilled chicken skewers. Also try it as a "lettuce stuffer" for a sandwich-like appetizer (or lunch!).

2 eggplants (about 2¾ pounds total), peeled, quartered, and chopped into big pieces

½ cup water, divided

3 teaspoons kosher salt

⅓ cup fresh lemon juice (about 2 lemons worth)

2 tablespoons extra-virgin olive oil

⅓ cup tahini

4 cloves fresh garlic, minced

¾ cup chopped fresh parsley

¼ teaspoon Tabasco sauce (about 2 shakes)

1. Place eggplant pieces in slow cooker crock and toss with the salt. Add 2 tablespoons of the water; cover and cook on LOW for 6 hours.

2. Remove eggplant to a food processor; add lemon juice and olive oil, then pulse to combine. Add all remaining ingredients to the food processor except the remaining water and blend until smooth. Continue to blend, adding water if necessary, until it reaches the consistency you desire.

3. Chill the babaghanoush overnight, to allow flavors to blend. Ideally, this dish is served at room temperature, so remove it from the refrigerator an hour before serving, if possible.

approximate nutritional content
▶ Calories: 66, Protein: 2g, Net Carbs: 4g, Fat: 4g, Cholesterol: 0mg, Sodium: 95mg

▶ **cook's tip**

Use fresh lemon juice and garlic in this dish; it really makes a difference! To get the most juice from your lemons, microwave them on HIGH for 35 seconds before juicing them.

con queso dip

▶ **ESTIMATED PREPARATION TIME:** 5 minutes ▶ **COOK TIME:** 2 hours in mini slow cooker ▶ **SERVINGS:** 8

This recipe was developed using a mini slow cooker (1¾ cups capacity) made by Rival. To double the recipe for a crowd, just use a larger slow cooker and cook on LOW.

8 ounces Velveeta, cut into 1-inch cubes
1 4-ounce can chopped green chilies
¼ teaspoon chili powder
¼ teaspoon black pepper
2 tablespoons low-carb beer
½ cup shredded cheddar cheese

1. Place Velveeta in the slow cooker crock; top with remaining ingredients.
2. Cover and cook for 1 hour. Uncover and stir to combine ingredients. Continue to cook 1 hour more (uncovered), stirring several times.

approximate nutritional content
 ▶ Calories: 117, Protein: 7g, Net Carbs: 4g, Fat: 8g, Cholesterol: 28mg, Sodium: 482mg

▶ **serving suggestion**
Serve with ready-made low-carb tortilla chips and red and green bell pepper strips.

creamy bacon-horseradish dip

▶ **ESTIMATED PREPARATION TIME:** 5 minutes   ▶ **COOK TIME:** 2 hours in mini slow cooker   ▶ **SERVINGS:** 16

Serve this and some Buttered Roasted Almonds (page 136) and they'll be talking about your party 'round the water cooler come Monday morning! If you're having company over, just double the recipe and use a larger slow cooker (be sure to cook on LOW). —KM

⅓ cup bacon pieces (about 3 slices, cooked and chopped)

1 cup cream cheese, softened in microwave for 45 seconds

⅓ cup bottled ranch dressing

3 tablespoons prepared horseradish

2 slices American cheese, chopped roughly

⅛ teaspoon black pepper

¼ teaspoon Tabasco sauce (about 2 shakes)

3 scallions, thinly sliced (optional)

1. Mix all ingredients together in a medium mixing bowl. Transfer mixture to the slow cooker crock.

2. Cover and cook for 2 hours, stirring once during cooking, and again at the end of cooking time. Top with sliced scallions before serving, if desired.

approximate nutritional content
▶ Calories: 89, Protein: 72g, Net Carbs: 1g, Fat: 9g, Cholesterol: 22mg, Sodium: 124mg

▶ **cook's tip**
Leftover dip makes a great spread for low-carb tortillas; add some turkey and lettuce and call it lunch!

▶ **serving suggestion**
Serve with ready-made low-carb crackers and plenty of fresh vegetables.

easy cheese dip

▶ **ESTIMATED PREPARATION TIME:** 5 minutes ▶ **COOK TIME:** 2 hours in a mini slow cooker ▶ **SERVINGS:** 12

My friend Mary Jo Chapman gave me this versatile cheese dip recipe. If you want a lot of cheese dip, just double the recipe and use a larger slow cooker set to LOW. —KM

8 ounces Velveeta, cut into 1-inch cubes
½ cup half-and-half
¼ cup shredded reduced-fat cheddar cheese
4 ounces "lite" cream cheese
¼ teaspoon Tabasco sauce (about 2 shakes)

1. Place all ingredients into the slow cooker.
2. Cover and cook for 1 hour. Stir the dip and cook for 1 hour more. Stir again prior to serving.

approximate nutritional content
▶ Calories: 99, Protein: 5g, Net Carbs: 3g, Fat: 8g, Cholesterol: 26mg, Sodium: 346mg

EASY ADD-IN

Create a Bacon Cheese Dip by adding ¼ cup chopped bacon pieces and ¼ teaspoon black pepper. The approximate nutritional content of this recipe is:
▶ Calories: 105, Protein: 6g, Net Carbs: 4g, Fat: 8g, Cholesterol: 27mg, Sodium: 363mg

▶ **serving suggestion**
Serve with ready-made low-carb tortilla chips or low-carb crackers and raw vegetables.

easy cheese and spinach dip

▶ **ESTIMATED PREPARATION TIME:** 10 minutes   ▶ **COOK TIME:** 2 hours   ▶ **SERVINGS:** 12

This variation of Easy Cheese Dip (page 146) is perfect for those times when you want a more substantial or more "special" dip. This dip is especially good with a raw vegetable platter. Unlike most of our other dip recipes, you'll need at least a 3-quart slow cooker (or larger, if you want to double the recipe) to prepare it.

8 ounces Velveeta, cut into 1-inch cubes
½ cup half-and-half
¼ cup shredded reduced-fat cheddar cheese
4 ounces "lite" cream cheese
¼ teaspoon Tabasco sauce (about 2 shakes)
1 teaspoon black pepper
1 tablespoon dried minced onions
1 10-ounce package chopped frozen spinach (thawed, with all water pressed out)
½ cup sliced black olives

1. Place all ingredients, except for the black olives, into the slow cooker crock.
2. Cover and cook on LOW for 1 hour. Stir the dip; cook on LOW for 1 hour more.
3. When done cooking, stir in black olives.

approximate nutritional content
▶ Calories: 110, Protein: 6g, Net Carbs: 4g, Fat: 9g, Cholesterol: 26mg, Sodium: 406mg

onion and spinach dip

▶ **ESTIMATED PREPARATION TIME:** 5 minutes ▶ **COOK TIME:** 2 hours in a mini slow cooker ▶ **SERVINGS:** 10

If you have a larger slow cooker and want to make a larger quantity of dip, just double the ingredients and cook on LOW.

1 packet dry onion soup mix

1 cup mayonnaise

⅓ cup "lite" cream cheese

½ cup chopped frozen spinach, thawed and squeezed dry

pinch kosher salt

½ teaspoon pepper

½ teaspoon Worcestershire sauce

¼ teaspoon Tabasco sauce (about 2 shakes)

1. Place all ingredients into the slow cooker crock.
2. Cover and cook on LOW for 1 hour. Stir the dip and cook 1 hour more. Stir again prior to serving.

approximate nutritional content
▶ Calories: 178, Protein: 1g, Net Carbs: 2g, Fat: 19g, Cholesterol: 17mg, Sodium: 239mg

super crab dip

▶ **ESTIMATED PREPARATION TIME:** 10 minutes ▶ **COOK TIME:** 2 hours in mini slow cooker ▶ **SERVINGS:** 12

This recipe makes about 1½ cups of dip—not much really, considering how delicious it is. Therefore, if you're having a party and don't have a mini slow cooker, not a problem—just double the recipe and make it in your larger machine (cook on LOW). Don't worry, there won't be leftovers!

¾ cup mayonnaise

1 teaspoon Worcestershire sauce

1 teaspoon soy sauce

¼ teaspoon black pepper

¼ teaspoon Tabasco sauce (about 2 shakes)

¼ teaspoon kosher salt

2 teaspoons fresh lemon juice

4 ounces cream cheese, very soft (heat in the microwave briefly, to soften, if necessary)

2 6-ounce cans crab meat, water pressed out

1. In a small mixing bowl, combine all ingredients except the crab; blend well with a whisk. Stir in the crab gently with a spoon.
2. Transfer mixture to the slow cooker crock and cook for 2 hours.

approximate nutritional content
▶ Calories: 156, Protein: 6g, Net Carbs: 1g, Fat: 15g, Cholesterol: 40mg, Sodium: 229mg

EASY ADD-IN
If you'd like a spicier dip, add 1 tablespoon prepared horseradish.

> ▶ **party planning tip**
> This dip can be made the night before and reheated, for a party.

cocktail party meatballs

▶ **ESTIMATED PREPARATION TIME:** 5 minutes ▶ **COOK TIME:** 4 hours ▶ **SERVINGS:** 15

Meatballs are always one of the first things to go at a party, and these will be no exception. To avoid running out, consider doubling the recipe.

1 green bell pepper, finely chopped
1 red bell pepper, finely chopped
1 tablespoon minced garlic
½ cup Splenda Granular sweetener
½ cup red wine vinegar
1 tablespoon soy sauce
2 tablespoons quick-cooking tapioca
½ teaspoon kosher salt
½ teaspoon black pepper
2 teaspoons dried minced onions
¾ cup water
2 tablespoons tomato paste
1 tablespoon Dijon mustard
1 2-pound bag frozen prepared meatballs, thawed

1. Add all ingredients except the meatballs to the slow cooker crock. Mix well, then add meatballs and stir to coat them with the sauce.
2. Cover and cook on LOW for 4 hours, stirring 2 or 3 times during cooking.

approximate nutritional content
  ▶ Calories: 76, Protein: 3g, Net Carbs: 10g, Fat: 3g, Cholesterol: 4mg, Sodium: 349mg

---

▶ **party planning tip**

If you're going to prepare two slow cooked foods for your party, plan on making one of the recipes the day before, and reheating it just before your guests arrive. Good choices for the do-ahead dish are the dips, which microwave nicely. Then you can use your slow cooker to prepare these meatballs (or any of the other party foods). You can even serve the meatballs directly from the slow cooker crock—saves dishes and time, and makes you look so clever!

---

chicken satay bites

▶ **ESTIMATED PREPARATION TIME:** 5 minutes (plus 8-12 hours marinating time) ▶ **COOK TIME:** 3 hours ▶ **SERVINGS:** 10

An exotic alternative to party meatballs. Your guests will appreciate the variety!

for the marinade:
2 tablespoons minced garlic
1 cup canned coconut milk
2 tablespoons bottled fish sauce
2 tablespoons red Thai curry paste
2 pounds skinless, boneless chicken breast, fat trimmed, cut into bite-sized pieces
2 tablespoons quick-cooking tapioca

for the peanut sauce:
½ cup bottled Thai peanut dipping sauce
¼ cup warm water
3 tablespoons smooth peanut butter

1. Whisk together the marinade ingredients in a small bowl. Pour mixture into a large zip-top bag; add chicken pieces, seal bag, and shake gently to coat chicken with marinade. Place the bag into the refrigerator and let marinate 8 to 12 hours (overnight is fine).

2. When done, drain off marinade and discard it. Place chicken pieces into the slow cooker crock. Add tapioca and stir to combine.

3. Cover and cook on LOW for 3 hours. When done, stir in the Thai peanut sauce, warm water, and peanut butter. Cover and cook about 15 minutes, or until sauce is heated through.

approximate nutritional content
▶ Calories: 252, Protein: 27g, Net Carbs: 6g, Fat: 13g, Cholesterol: 68mg, Sodium: 187mg

> ▶ **about the ingredients**
> We prefer the Thai Kitchen brand of bottled Thai ingredients such as the peanut sauce and curry paste. This brand is available in the "ethnic" section of many grocery stores. A comparable brand will work just fine.

meatballs stroganoff

▶ **ESTIMATED PREPARATION TIME:** 10 minutes ▶ **COOK TIME:** 4 hours ▶ **SERVINGS:** 15

This is a great party appetizer that puts all the flavors of beef stroganoff into a bite-sized, easy-to-eat form. Your guests will love these!

½ teaspoon black pepper

2 cubes beef bouillon

1 cup water

1 packet dry stroganoff sauce mix

2 tablespoons dried minced onions

1 10-ounce package of mushrooms, finely chopped

1 2-pound bag frozen prepared meatballs, thawed

1½ cups sour cream, room temperature

¼ teaspoon Tabasco sauce (about 2 shakes)

1. Add first 6 ingredients (pepper through mushrooms) to the slow cooker crock and mix well. Add the meatballs.
2. Cover and cook on LOW for 3 hours. Stir to coat meatballs with sauce, then cook 1 hour more.
3. Just before serving, add sour cream and Tabasco sauce; stir well.

approximate nutritional content
▶ Calories: 67, Protein: 12g, Net Carbs: 8g, Fat: 18g, Cholesterol: 48mg, Sodium: 576mg

▶ **party planning tip**
Don't forget to have plenty of toothpicks on hand when serving slow cooker appetizers such as meatballs or cocktail franks. Small plates are also essential, as people may want to serve themselves several meatballs at one time!

sweet-and-sour cocktail sausages

▶ **ESTIMATED PREPARATION TIME:** 5 minutes ▶ **COOK TIME:** 4 hours ▶ **SERVINGS:** 12

A low-carb version of a popular potluck dish. Easy and delicious!

1 6-ounce can tomato paste

⅓ cup red wine vinegar

½ teaspoon Worcestershire sauce

⅔ cup Splenda Granular sweetener

1 teaspoon black pepper

¾ teaspoon seasoning salt

½ teaspoon black pepper

⅔ cup water

¼ cup low-sugar grape jelly

3 16-ounce packages cocktail sausages

1. Add all ingredients, except the sausages, to the slow cooker crock. Mix until well-blended. Add sausages and stir to coat with sauce.

2. Cover and cook on LOW for 4 hours, stirring twice during cooking.

approximate nutritional content
▶ Calories: 371, Protein: 15g, Net Carbs: 7.5g, Fat: 32g, Cholesterol: 74mg, Sodium: 1,359mg

EASY SUBSTITUTION

If preferred, substitute cocktail wieners for the sausages.

▶ **party planning tip**

When considering how many appetizers to serve at a party, plan on each guest eating 3 to 5 pieces of each item, depending on how many appetizers you're serving. If you have only a few items to choose from, you'll need larger quantities of them. If you have a lavish spread, you won't need as many of each item. Consider, too, whether you'll be serving just appetizers or will follow them with a meal. If no meal will follow, make some of the appetizers "heavier," so guests won't go hungry!

cocktail sausages with low-carb bbq sauce

▶ **ESTIMATED PREPARATION TIME:** 10 minutes   ▶ **COOK TIME:** 4 hours   ▶ **SERVINGS:** 12

The perfect low-carb party fare. No one will know the difference!

1 6-ounce can tomato paste

⅓ cup white vinegar

¼ cup Splenda Granular sweetener

1 teaspoon black pepper

¾ teaspoon kosher salt

2 tablespoons Worcestershire sauce

½ teaspoon onion powder

½ teaspoon garlic powder

½ teaspoon paprika

½ teaspoon chili powder

¼ teaspoon minced fresh ginger

1 tablespoon brown mustard

1 cup water

1 tablespoon butter

3 16-ounce packages cocktail sausages

1. Add all ingredients, except the sausages, to the slow cooker crock. Mix until well-blended. Add sausages and stir to coat with sauce.

2. Cover and cook on LOW for 4 hours, stirring twice during cooking, and again before serving.

approximate nutritional content
▶ Calories: 375, Protein: 15g, Net Carbs: 5g, Fat: 33g, Cholesterol: 76mg, Sodium: 1,370mg

---

▶ **party planning tip**
This recipe can be made one day ahead, then reheated and transferred to a serving dish for the party. Or, make it 4 hours prior to the party, then serve right from your slow cooker (no extra dishes to wash!).

sweet-and-sour kielbasa slices

▶ **ESTIMATED PREPARATION TIME:** 10 minutes   ▶ **COOK TIME:** 6 hours   ▶ **SERVINGS:** 12

No one will guess this is low-carb, they'll just nosh happily.

1 green bell pepper, finely chopped

1 red bell pepper, finely chopped

2 teaspoons minced garlic

½ cup Splenda Granular sweetener

½ cup red wine vinegar

1 tablespoon soy sauce

2 tablespoons quick-cooking tapioca

¼ teaspoon black pepper

¼ teaspoon kosher salt

¼ teaspoon Tabasco sauce (about 2 shakes)

¼ teaspoon crushed red pepper flakes

1 teaspoon onion powder

¼ cup water

2 pounds kielbasa or "lite" kielbasa, sliced ¼-inch thick

1. Add all ingredients, except the kielbasa, to the slow cooker crock; mix well. Add kielbasa and stir to coat with sauce.
2. Cover and cook on LOW for 6 hours, stirring several times during cooking.

approximate nutritional content
▶ Calories: 246, Protein: 10g, Net Carbs: 5g, Fat: 21g, Cholesterol: 51mg, Sodium: 911mg

EASY SUBSTITUTION

If preferred, substitute cocktail sausages for the kielbasa. Doing so will change the approximate nutritional content to:
▶ Calories: 244, Protein: 10g, Net Carbs: 5g, Fat: 21g, Cholesterol: 49mg, Sodium: 869mg

crepesagna

▶ **ESTIMATED PREPARATION TIME:** 25 minutes ▶ **COOK TIME:** 3 hours ▶ **SERVINGS:** 8

Miss lasagna? Having a couple of friends over for dinner? Serve this special dish and they'll be amazed at your culinary creativity. Be aware that the carb content of this dish is higher than our typical recipe, so keep it for special occasions.

for the sauce:
2 tablespoons olive oil
1 medium onion, finely chopped
1 pound ground pork
1 pound ground veal or ground beef (90% lean)
¼ cup half-and-half
2 teaspoons oregano
¼ teaspoon black pepper
¼ teaspoon kosher salt
1 teaspoon minced garlic
1 26-ounce can "lite" or "no sugar added" spaghetti sauce

for the filling:
16 ounces part-skim ricotta cheese
1 egg, beaten
½ teaspoon kosher salt
¼ teaspoon black pepper
¼ cup grated Parmesan cheese
½ cup shredded part-skim mozzarella cheese

cooking spray
2 cups shredded part-skim mozzarella cheese, divided
4 ready-made crepes

1. Prepare the sauce: In a large skillet, over medium heat, warm olive oil; add onion and meats and cook thoroughly; drain the fat. Add the half-and-half and spices; mix well and simmer for 5 minutes. Add the spaghetti sauce and simmer another 10 minutes.

2. While sauce is simmering, mix together the filling ingredients in a medium bowl. Remove sauce from heat. Coat the slow cooker crock with cooking spray.

3. Assemble Crepesagna: Add 1 cup sauce to slow cooker and top with a crepe; drop ⅓ cup ricotta mixture by small spoonfuls on top of crepe, top with ½ cup mozzarella cheese, and pour 2 cups meat sauce over. Then start with another crepe and repeat the process two more times, ending with a crepe and the last of the mozzarella.

4. Cover and cook on LOW for 3 hours. Turn off slow cooker and let Crepesagna rest, uncovered, for 15 minutes before serving.

approximate nutritional content
▶ Calories: 585, Protein: 47g, Net Carbs: 21g, Fat: 33g, Cholesterol: 234mg, Sodium: 880mg

---

▶ **about the ingredients**
Crepes are a decent substitute for pasta. Although they don't taste exactly like pasta, they do keep the fillings separate and help give this recipe structure. They are typically found near the berries in the produce section of the grocery store.

---

double-duty recipes

corned beef and cabbage

▶ **ESTIMATED PREPARATION TIME:** 10 minutes ▶ **COOK TIME:** 10 hours ▶ **SERVINGS:** 6

Unless you're serving six at your table, you'll have meat leftover to prepare Corned Beef and Onion Hash (page 159) tomorrow! This dish will get your low-carb Irish eyes smiling. —KM

1 tablespoon butter
1 medium onion, halved and thinly sliced
1 pound baby carrots
½ head cabbage (about 1½ pounds), cored and cut into 1-inch slices
1 cube beef bouillon
½ teaspoon kosher salt
1 teaspoon black pepper
1 tablespoon minced garlic
2 cups white wine
4-pound corned beef brisket, fat trimmed

1. Place the butter in the bottom of the slow cooker crock, then layer the onions, then the carrots, and finally the cabbage on top. Add the bouillon, salt, pepper, garlic, and white wine. Top with the corned beef and pour water over all, being sure beef is covered with water. The pot will be very full.

2. Cover and cook on LOW for 10 hours. Let the corned beef sit, uncovered, for 15 minutes before slicing and serving.

3. To serve, slice corned beef across the grain into thin slices. Remove vegetables from the slow cooker using a slotted spoon, and serve alongside the corned beef.

approximate nutritional content
▶ Calories: 477, Protein: 28g, Net Carbs: 12g, Fat: 28g, Cholesterol: 140mg, Sodium: 1,805mg

▶ **cook's tip**
Buy a "flat-cut" corned beef—it's a better-quality cut.

▶ **serving suggestion**
Serve with toasted, low-carb rye bread, and a good-quality mustard for the beef. Low-carb beer optional!

corned beef and onion hash

▶ **ESTIMATED PREPARATION TIME:** 5 minutes ▶ **COOK TIME:** 15 minutes ▶ **SERVINGS:** 5

Hash is always a welcome change at the breakfast table, and it makes a great supper, too. If you don't have leftover corned beef from Corned Beef and Cabbage (page 158), then buy some corned beef at the deli counter.

3 tablespoons butter

½ red onion, finely chopped

1 cup frozen cauliflower, thawed and finely chopped

1½ teaspoons black pepper

½ teaspoon kosher salt

½ teaspoon garlic powder

2 teaspoons dried minced onions

1 pound corned beef, finely chopped, or shredded in a food processor (about 3 cups)

1. In a large, nonstick skillet, melt the butter over medium-low heat; add the red onions, cauliflower, pepper, salt, garlic, and dried onions; cook 10 minutes, stirring, until onions are very soft. Add the corned beef and cook another 5 minutes, until mixture is sizzling.

2. Stir mixture, adding 1 tablespoon water to loosen mixture from the bottom of the skillet, if necessary. Serve hot.

approximate nutritional content
▶ Calories: 305, Protein: 18g, Net Carbs: 3g, Fat: 24g, Cholesterol: 108mg, Sodium: 1,154mg

▶ **serving suggestion**
This is scrumptious served with an egg or two and buttered, low-carb toast.

double-duty recipes **159**

chicken with 40 cloves of garlic

▶ **ESTIMATED PREPARATION TIME:** 10 minutes ▶ **COOK TIME:** 9 hours ▶ **SERVINGS:** 5

Don't let the amount of garlic scare you! This is a classic French dish that's nicely suited to slow cooking. The garlic softens and develops a milder, sweet flavor during cooking. We used a large chicken specifically to get leftovers for Classic Chicken Salad (page 161) and Dijon Ranch Chicken Salad (page 163). However, you can easily adapt this recipe for a smaller bird (3–4 pounds) by halving the ingredient amounts and using a 4-quart slow cooker.

2 teaspoons ground thyme
2 tablespoons olive oil
½ teaspoon black pepper
½ teaspoon kosher salt
6- to 7-pound roasting chicken, rinsed, with giblets and neck removed
40 whole, peeled garlic cloves
2 tablespoons white wine

1. Add the first four ingredients to the slow cooker crock and stir to combine. Place the chicken in the crock and roll it around and flip it over to coat with the oil mixture. Place ½ of the garlic (20 cloves) inside the cavity of the bird. Make sure bird is placed breast-side down in the slow cooker crock.

2. Sprinkle remaining garlic around the chicken. Pour the wine down the side of the crock and into the bottom (not over the chicken itself).

3. Cover and cook on LOW for 8 hours. Check chicken for doneness using an instant-read thermometer (it should register 170°F). If it's done, let the bird rest, covered, in the slow cooker crock for 15 minutes. If the chicken has not reached 170°F, cook another hour, then recheck the temperature.

approximate nutritional content
▶ Calories: 537, Protein: 74g, Net Carbs: 0.5g, Fat: 24g, Cholesterol: 227mg, Sodium: 267mg

▶ **cook's tip**
Peeling garlic is labor-intensive, but you can skip this step by purchasing whole, peeled garlic cloves in a jar in your supermarket's produce section (perhaps next to the fresh garlic and onions).

▶ **serving suggestion**
This chicken is wonderful served with Warm Spinach Salad (page 197).

classic chicken salad

▶ **ESTIMATED PREPARATION TIME:** 3 minutes ▶ **COOK TIME:** none ▶ **SERVINGS:** 2

If you're craving a chicken salad sandwich, this is the filling you're looking for. Use leftover meat from Chicken with 40 Cloves of Garlic (page 160) for its delicious garlic flavor.

2 cups cooked chicken meat, chopped
4 scallions, thinly sliced
1 tablespoon lemon juice
¼ cup mayonnaise
⅛ teaspoon kosher salt
¼ teaspoon black pepper
¼ teaspoon Tabasco sauce (about 2 shakes)

1. In a medium mixing bowl, stir together all ingredients. Refrigerate if not using immediately.

approximate nutritional content
▶ Calories: 471, Protein: 41g, Net Carbs: 2g, Fat: 32g, Cholesterol: 141mg, Sodium: 319mg

toasted-walnut and apple chicken salad

▶ **ESTIMATED PREPARATION TIME:** 10 minutes (includes toasting walnuts) ▶ **COOK TIME:** none ▶ **SERVINGS:** 3

This is a slightly sweeter, crunchier version of Classic Chicken Salad (page 161). Note the increased number of portions with this variation.

½ cup walnuts, chopped and toasted

½ medium apple, cored and chopped

2 cups cooked chicken meat, chopped

4 scallions, thinly sliced

1 tablespoon lemon juice

¼ cup mayonnaise

⅛ teaspoon kosher salt

¼ teaspoon black pepper

¼ teaspoon Tabasco sauce (about 2 shakes)

1. In a medium mixing bowl, stir together all ingredients. Refrigerate if not using immediately.

approximate nutritional content
   ▶ Calories: 456, Protein: 30g, Net Carbs: 7g, Fat: 34g, Cholesterol: 94mg, Sodium: 215mg

dijon ranch chicken salad

▶ **ESTIMATED PREPARATION TIME:** 10 minutes (includes toasting almonds) ▶ **COOK TIME:** none ▶ **SERVINGS:** 2

Chicken salad is an easy and delicious way to use up leftover chicken meat from a previously slow-cooked dish, such as Chicken with 40 Cloves of Garlic (page 160).

2 cups cooked chicken meat, chopped

5 radishes, finely chopped

1 stalk celery, finely chopped

¼ cup red onion, finely chopped

1½ tablespoons prepared Dijon mustard

1 tablespoon mayonnaise

3 tablespoons bottled ranch dressing

⅓ cup sliced almonds, toasted

⅛ teaspoon black pepper

1. In a medium mixing bowl, stir together all ingredients. Refrigerate if not using immediately.

approximate nutritional content
   ▶ Calories: 508, Protein: 45g, Net Carbs: 6g, Fat: 32g, Cholesterol: 138mg, Sodium: 563mg

▶ **serving suggestion**

This chicken salad is especially nice served atop a big plate of green salad for a light dinner. Or, wrap ¼ to ½ cup of chicken salad mixture in large lettuce leaves for roll-ups.

overnight hard-boiled eggs

▶ **ESTIMATED PREPARATION TIME:** 1 minute ▶ **COOK TIME:** 8 hours ▶ **SERVINGS:** 18 eggs

Let your slow cooker do the work while you're sleeping! You'll have plenty of hard-boiled eggs on hand for snacking, salad toppers, and for making Classic Egg Salad (page 165).

18 white eggs
water

1. Check the eggs for hairline cracks and discard those eggs. Gently place remaining eggs into the slow cooker crock and add cold water to cover them.
2. Cover and cook on LOW for 8 hours. After cooking, gently remove the hard-boiled eggs to a bowl and run cold water over them until cool; store in the refrigerator.

approximate nutritional content
▶ Calories: 78, Protein: 6g, Net Carbs: 0.5g, Fat: 5g, Cholesterol: 212mg, Sodium: 62mg

▶ **cook's tip**
You may want to mark your hard-boiled eggs with a pencil (after cooking) to help you tell them apart from your regular eggs. Or, keep them in a covered bowl, separate from your other eggs.

▶ **about the ingredients**
White-shelled eggs are the best choice for this recipe. Be aware that the whites of the eggs will turn a light beige color during slow cooking. However, if you use brown-shelled eggs, the whites will turn very beige, and while the flavor is unaffected, you may find the color unappealing.

classic egg salad

▶ **ESTIMATED PREPARATION TIME:** 5 minutes   ▶ **COOK TIME:** none (uses precooked eggs)   ▶ **SERVINGS:** 4

This old favorite makes a great salad topper or filling for a large lettuce leaf.

½ cup mayonnaise (or reduced-calorie mayonnaise)

1 tablespoon brown or yellow prepared mustard

¼ teaspoon black pepper

pinch kosher salt

8 hard-boiled eggs, peeled and chopped

1. In a medium mixing bowl, combine all ingredients, except the eggs, and stir together well. Add chopped eggs and stir gently to combine. Refrigerate if not using immediately.

approximate nutritional content
▶ Calories: 358, Protein: 13g, Net Carbs: 2g, Fat: 33g, Cholesterol: 440mg, Sodium: 399mg

pickled eggs

▶ **ESTIMATED PREPARATION TIME:** 5 minutes   ▶ **COOK TIME:** none (refrigerate at least 3 days)   ▶ **SERVINGS:** 6

New ways to prepare eggs are always welcome in a low-carb household!

¾ cup water
¾ cup white vinegar
1 clove garlic, halved
½ teaspoon pickling spice
½ teaspoon pickling salt
1½ teaspoons dried minced onions
1 tablespoon Splenda Granular sweetener
6 hard-boiled eggs, peeled

1. In a clean large glass jar (such as a mayonnaise jar), mix together all ingredients, except for the eggs.
2. Carefully place eggs, one at a time, into the jar of seasoning liquid. Cover jar and refrigerate eggs at least 3 days.

approximate nutritional content
▶ Calories: 83, Protein: 6g, Net Carbs: 3g, Fat: 5g, Cholesterol: 212mg, Sodium: 102mg

---

▶ **about the ingredients**

Confused about pickling salt versus regular salt versus kosher salt? Pickling salt lacks the iodine and anticaking additives that regular table salt contains. Kosher salt contains no iodine but may contain yellow prussiate of soda, an anticaking agent. Foods pickled with regular table salt would still be good to eat, but they wouldn't look as appetizing, because the additives tend to turn the pickled foods dark and the pickling liquid cloudy. Pickling salt is available in large boxes in supermarkets, although it can be hard to find in cities. If you can't find pickling salt, use kosher salt (it won't turn the pickles dark). Be aware, however, that because the grains of kosher salt are flakier than pickling salt, it doesn't measure exactly like pickling salt. Therefore, if you're using kosher salt in this recipe, use slightly more than ½ teaspoon, but not quite ¾ teaspoon.

spicy pickled eggs

▶ **ESTIMATED PREPARATION TIME:** 5 minutes ▶ **COOK TIME:** none (refrigerate at least 3 days) ▶ **SERVINGS:** 6

These will give your taste buds a wake-up call! Guests will love them, too.

1 cup white vinegar
2 tablespoons minced garlic
2 teaspoons red pepper flakes
2 cups water
1 tablespoon pickling salt
6 hard-boiled eggs, peeled

1. In a clean large glass jar (such as a mayonnaise jar), mix together all ingredients, except for the eggs.
2. Carefully place eggs, one at a time, into the jar of seasoning liquid. Cover jar and refrigerate eggs at least 3 days.

approximate nutritional content
▶ Calories: 84, Protein: 7g, Net Carbs: 2g, Fat: 5g, Cholesterol: 212mg, Sodium: 1,129mg

smoked picnic ham with cabbage

▶ **ESTIMATED PREPARATION TIME:** 5 minutes ▶ **COOK TIME:** 9 hours ▶ **SERVINGS:** 6

An easy family favorite that yields plenty of leftover meat (about 3 cups) to use in a batch of Ham, Spinach, and White Bean Soup (page 169).

cooking spray

5- to 6-pound smoked shoulder picnic ham

2 tablespoons white wine

2 tablespoons water

1 tablespoon brown mustard

¼ teaspoon black pepper

1 small head of green cabbage, cored and cut into wedges (or ½ of a large cabbage)

1 medium onion, halved and sliced

1. Coat the slow cooker crock with cooking spray. Add the wine, water, mustard, and pepper to the crock and stir until blended.

2. Add half of the cabbage wedges and half the onion slices to the crock; toss to coat with the wine mixture. Top with the ham and place the remaining cabbage and onions around the ham.

3. Cover and cook on LOW for 8½ hours. Stir the cabbage (around the ham) so the cabbage gets coated with cooking juices; cook another ½ hour more.

approximate nutritional content

▶ Calories: 581, Protein: 50g, Net Carbs: 2.5g, Fat: 39g, Cholesterol: 141mg, Sodium: 2,731mg

ham, spinach, and white bean soup

▶ **PREPARATION TIME:** 15 minutes ▶ **COOKING TIME:** 6 hours ▶ **SERVINGS:** 6

This is a great way to use up leftover ham from the Smoked Picnic Ham with Cabbage (page 168). Plus, your whole family will enjoy this healthy, hearty soup. It freezes well, so keep a little aside for a quick lunch later.

cooking spray

3 cups cooked ham, cubed (about 1½ pounds)

1 10-ounce package frozen chopped spinach, thawed

½ pound (½ bag) frozen cauliflower, thawed and chopped

2 celery stalks, sliced in half lengthwise and finely chopped

1 medium onion, finely chopped

6 cups chicken stock

2 cups water

½ teaspoon black pepper

1 15.5-ounce can small white beans (such as Great Northern beans), rinsed and drained

½ teaspoon Tabasco sauce (about 4 shakes)

1. Coat the slow cooker crock with cooking spray. Add all ingredients to the crock, except for the beans and Tabasco sauce; gently stir to combine.

2. Cover and cook on LOW for 5½ to 6 hours. Stir in drained beans and Tabasco sauce, then cook ½ hour more. Taste before serving to determine if additional salt is needed (it probably won't be).

approximate nutritional content
▶ Calories: 304, Protein: 35g, Net Carbs: 11g, Fat: 11g, Cholesterol: 67mg, Sodium: 2,707mg

EASY SUBSTITUTION
Cooked chicken meat, cubed (3 cups), can be substituted for the ham. To do so, increase chicken stock to 8 cups and eliminate the water. This change will alter the approximate nutritional content to:
▶ Calories: 259, Protein: 27g, Net Carbs: 11g, Fat: 10g, Cholesterol: 68mg, Sodium: 1,263mg

cheesy mock mashed potatoes with sour cream

▶ **ESTIMATED PREPARATION TIME:** 5 minutes   ▶ **COOK TIME:** 4 hours   ▶ **SERVINGS:** 4 1-cup servings (plus 3 cups leftovers)

The leftovers from this recipe form the topping for Shepherd's Pie (page 171). In this recipe, we used regular cheese instead of reduced-fat, to enhance the richness of the finished dish. Feel free to substitute reduced-fat cheddar, if you like.

3 tablespoons butter

$\frac{1}{2}$ cup chicken broth

2 tablespoons quick-cooking tapioca

$\frac{1}{2}$ teaspoon kosher salt

$\frac{1}{2}$ teaspoon black pepper

2 1-pound bags frozen cauliflower

$\frac{1}{4}$ teaspoon Tabasco sauce (about 2 shakes)

6 ounces shredded white cheddar cheese (1$\frac{1}{2}$ cups)

1 cup sour cream

crumbled, cooked bacon pieces (optional)

1. Grease the slow cooker crock with the butter (leave excess in the crock). Add the broth, tapioca, salt, and pepper and mix well. Top mixture with the cauliflower, cover, and cook on LOW for 4 hours. (Cooking a little longer than this may result in some brown edges but will not hurt the flavor of the dish.)

2. After 4 hours, switch the slow cooker to WARM (if available; leave on LOW if not available), add the Tabasco sauce, cheese, and sour cream. Using a potato masher, mash all ingredients together in the slow cooker crock.

3. Serve warm, garnished with crumbled bacon pieces, if desired.

approximate nutritional content
▶ Calories: 257, Protein: 10g, Net Carbs: 8.5g, Fat: 20g, Cholesterol: 54mg, Sodium: 365mg

shepherd's pie

▶ **ESTIMATED PREPARATION TIME:** 15 minutes ▶ **COOK TIME:** 35–45 minutes in oven ▶ **SERVINGS:** 6

Using leftover cheesy Mock Mashed Potatoes with sour cream (page 170) makes this family favorite a snap to prepare. Note that the carb content of this recipe is higher than usual for this book; therefore, keep this recipe for a special occasion.

cooking spray
1½ pounds lean ground beef (90% lean)
1 tablespoon dried minced onions
1 packet brown gravy mix
1 teaspoon black pepper
¼ teaspoon kosher salt
1 14.5-ounce can creamed corn
3 cups leftover Cheesy Mock Mashed
   Potatoes
⅛ teaspoon paprika

1. Preheat oven to 350°F. Coat a 10-inch pie plate or round cake pan with cooking spray; set aside.
2. In a large skillet, over medium-high heat, brown the ground beef until cooked through. Add dried onions, gravy mix, pepper, and salt to the skillet and stir well to combine. Transfer beef mixture to the greased pie plate.
3. Top the beef layer with the creamed corn, then spread the Cheesy Mock Mashed Potatoes over the corn for a final layer. Sprinkle with paprika and place pie pan on a baking sheet (in case it boils over).
4. Bake pie for 35 to 45 minutes. Remove from oven and let pie cool 5 to 10 minutes before serving.

approximate nutritional content
▶ Calories: 452, Protein: 35g, Net Carbs: 21g, Fat: 26g, Cholesterol: 128mg, Sodium: 637mg

thanksgiving anytime turkey breast

▶ **ESTIMATED PREPARATION TIME:** 10 minutes   ▶ **COOK TIME:** 8 hours   ▶ **SERVINGS:** 8

For those days when you want the taste of Thanksgiving without all the fuss! Unless you're serving a crowd, you'll have leftovers. Use them in the classic way: turkey sandwiches. Our BLT Sandwich (page 173)—bacon, lettuce, and turkey—is a delicious choice.

cooking spray
2 tablespoons white wine
½ cup chicken broth
1 onion, thinly sliced
4 cloves garlic, each sliced in half
6- to 8-pound "hotel" turkey breast
   (no legs or thighs), giblets removed,
   rinsed and dried
¾ teaspoon celery salt
½ teaspoon black pepper
½ teaspoon paprika

1. Coat the slow cooker crock with cooking spray. Add the wine, broth, onion, and garlic pieces.
2. Place the turkey breast, neck up (cavity opening facing down) in the slow cooker crock. Sprinkle turkey with the celery salt, pepper, and paprika, then spray over it with cooking spray.
3. Cook on LOW for 8 hours. Check for doneness using an instant read thermometer (it should register 170°F). If not done, cook an additional hour and check again.
4. Carefully remove the turkey breast from the crock, using two large forks. Let turkey rest on a platter or cutting board, covered with foil, for at least 5 minutes before slicing. Serve with Turkey au Jus "Gravy" (page 178), if desired.

approximate nutritional content (for plain turkey breast)
▶ Calories: 439, Protein: 65g, Net Carbs: 1g, Fat: 17g, Cholesterol: 170mg, Sodium: 415mg

blt sandwich (bacon, lettuce, and turkey)

▶ **ESTIMATED PREPARATION TIME:** 5 minutes ▶ **COOK TIME:** none ▶ **SERVINGS:** 2

A great way to use up leftover Thanksgiving Anytime Turkey Breast (page 172), this sandwich combines lots of favorite flavors.

4 slices low-carb bread, toasted

2 tablespoons mayonnaise

4 leaves iceberg lettuce

2 thin slices cheddar cheese (about 2 ounces total)

4 slices bacon, cooked

$\frac{1}{4}$ pound roasted turkey breast meat, sliced

salt and pepper to taste

1. Spread each piece of low–carb toast with $\frac{1}{2}$ tablespoon of mayonnaise. Lay a lettuce leaf on each piece of toast.
2. Top two of the pieces of toast with the cheddar, bacon, and turkey; sprinkle with salt and pepper. Finally, top with remaining two pieces of toast. Cut each sandwich and serve.

approximate nutritional content
▶ Calories: 527, Protein: 40g, Net Carbs: 16g, Fat: 34g, Cholesterol: 86mg, Sodium: 975mg

sauces, dressings, and toppings

meatballs and sauce

▶ **ESTIMATED PREPARATION TIME:** 15 minutes   ▶ **COOK TIME:** 8 hours   ▶ **SERVINGS:** 6

The meatballs cook right in the sauce, making it especially rich and robust. If
you like, serve with spaghetti squash (see below) or low-carb pasta.

for the meatballs:

1 pound ground pork

1 pound ground veal or lean ground beef
    (90% lean)

3 eggs, beaten

½ cup grated Parmesan cheese

1 tablespoon onion powder

2 teaspoons garlic powder

1 tablespoon oregano

¾ teaspoon kosher salt

1 teaspoon black pepper

for the sauce:

1 25.75-ounce can "lite" or "no sugar
    added" spaghetti sauce

2 teaspoons oregano

1 teaspoon minced garlic

½ teaspoon black pepper

2 teaspoons butter

¼ cup red wine

1 cup water

1. In a large mixing bowl, using clean hands, combine
   meatball ingredients; set aside. In slow cooker crock,
   whisk together the sauce ingredients.
2. Form meat mixture into golf ball–sized meatballs and
   drop them into the sauce (some will stick out of the
   sauce; that's okay).
3. Cover and cook on LOW for 8 hours. Before serving,
   stir gently so all meatballs are coated with sauce.

approximate nutritional content
   ▶ Calories: 365, Protein: 40g, Net Carbs: 10g, Fat: 16g,
   Cholesterol: 224mg, Sodium: 750mg

▶ **cook's tip**

To quickly cook a spaghetti squash, cut a small squash (about 2
pounds) in half lengthwise, scrape out seeds with a spoon, place
each half cut-side down in a microwaveable dish, add 2 cups
water and cover with microwavable plastic wrap. Microwave on
HIGH for 10 to 15 minutes (use a fork to check tenderness of
squash after 10 minutes). When done, let cool and scrape the
"spaghetti" out with a fork. This yields about 3 cups of "spaghetti,"
enough for 4 servings. Each serving of spaghetti squash contains
5g Net Carbs.

creamy cheese sauce

▶ **ESTIMATED PREPARATION TIME:** 1 minute   ▶ **COOK TIME:** 15 minutes   ▶ **SERVINGS:** 6

If you're making this sauce for the Chicken Cordon Bleu Roll-Ups (page 33), begin preparing
it when the roll-ups have finished cooking. With tongs, remove roll-ups to a plate and cover with foil
to keep warm while you're preparing the sauce. Even if you haven't made the roll-ups, you can make
this sauce to go over baked or roasted chicken and the like. Just make it on the stove top.

Remaining Swiss cheese from Chicken
  Cordon Bleu Roll-Ups, or about ½ cup
  chopped cheese
Remaining drippings from Chicken Cordon
  Bleu Roll-Ups (or about 1 cup broth)
1 cup heavy cream
¼ teaspoon black pepper
¼ teaspoon Tabasco sauce (about 2
  shakes)

1. In a medium saucepan, heat heavy cream over medium heat until reduced by half, about 10 to 12 minutes, stirring occasionally.
2. Meanwhile, turn slow cooker to HIGH, remove lid and heat drippings (broth) from roll-ups, until slightly reduced, about 5 minutes.
3. When cream is reduced, stir in black pepper and Tabasco sauce; pour in reduced drippings and Swiss cheese. Whisk until smooth and heated through. Pass sauce with roll-ups or pour it on top of roll-ups before serving.

approximate nutritional content
  ▶ Calories: 178, Protein: 4g, Net Carbs: 1g, Fat: 18g,
  Cholesterol: 63mg, Sodium: 206mg

turkey au jus "gravy"

▶ **ESTIMATED PREPARATION TIME:** 2 minutes ▶ **COOK TIME:** none ▶ **SERVINGS:** 6

A super-easy way to make a little "gravy" for your Thanksgiving Anytime Turkey Breast (page 172).

Remaining onion/garlic (about ¼ cup) from Thanksgiving Anytime Turkey Breast

Remaining liquid drippings (about 1½ cups broth) from Thanksgiving Anytime Turkey Breast

1. Using a hand blender, carefully blend the onions, garlic, and remaining drippings in the crock of the slow cooker. Serve hot.

2. Alternatively, a regular blender may be used to make the "gravy." To do so, skim onions and garlic out of the slow cooker and blend them with ½ cup of the liquid drippings. Be careful when transferring and blending liquid (leave the vent open on the blender to let steam escape), as it may still be very hot. When blended, add mixture back to remaining liquid drippings and stir to combine.

approximate nutritional content
▶ Calories: 13, Protein: 0g, Net Carbs: 0g, Fat: 1g, Cholesterol: 1mg, Sodium: 250mg

vegetable sauce

▶ **ESTIMATED PREPARATION TIME:** 15 minutes ▶ **COOK TIME:** 8 hours ▶ **SERVINGS:** 8

This sauce is so much more flavorful than anything you'll find in a jar at the grocery store! Take advantage of vegetables on special sale, or at your farmer's market, then make a batch of this sauce and freeze it for later use.

¼ cup olive oil

1 medium (about 1 pound) eggplant, peeled and cubed

½ pound fresh green beans, cut into 1-inch pieces

1 medium onion, finely chopped

1 7-ounce can sliced mushrooms

1 carrot, peeled and finely chopped

1 celery stalk, finely chopped

3 cups crushed tomatoes (either fresh or canned)

¼ cup red wine

1 teaspoon black pepper

1 teaspoon kosher salt

2 teaspoons oregano

2 tablespoons minced garlic

½ cup half-and-half

¼ teaspoon Tabasco sauce (about 2 shakes)

1. Brush the olive oil inside the slow cooker crock (leave excess in the crock). Add all ingredients except the half-and-half and Tabasco sauce to the crock and mix well.

2. Cover and cook on LOW for 8 hours. Before serving, mix in the half-and-half and the Tabasco sauce. Serve immediately, or freeze.

approximate nutritional content
   ▶ Calories: 152, Protein: 3g, Net Carbs: 9.5g, Fat: 9g, Cholesterol: 6mg, Sodium: 145mg

---

▶ **serving suggestions**

There are a variety of things you can do with this versatile sauce. Here are a few ideas:

■ Serve it over baked or grilled chicken breast

■ Serve it alongside broiled filet mignon

■ Use it as a "bed" for a grilled swordfish steak

■ Make a pasta sauce out of it (add about ¼ cup water to 1 cup of the sauce) and serve with low-carb pasta

buttered parmesan breadcrumbs

▶ **ESTIMATED PREPARATION TIME:** 5 minutes ▶ **COOK TIME:** 10 minutes ▶ **SERVINGS:** 2 cups (32 1-tablespoon servings)

Buttered breadcrumbs are a "secret weapon" of the Italian kitchen. They deliciously thicken sauces and soups, and also add a layer of flavor to veggies and pasta dishes. —KM

9 slices low-carb white bread, very stale
¼ cup butter
¼ teaspoon black pepper
¼ teaspoon kosher salt
½ cup grated Parmesan cheese
2 tablespoons dried parsley

1. Break up bread slices into a large zip-top bag. Using a rolling pin, crush the bread into crumbs. If you'd rather have very fine crumbs, chop the bread up in a food processor. Set breadcrumbs aside.

2. In a large skillet, over medium heat, melt the butter; add breadcrumbs, pepper, and salt. Cook until the crumbs smell toasty, about 5 minutes. Remove from heat and toss the crumbs, Parmesan, and parsley together in a large mixing bowl; let mixture cool.

3. Store in an airtight container until ready to use.

approximate nutritional content
▶ Calories: 38, Protein: 2g, Net Carbs: 1g, Fat: 2g, Cholesterol: 5mg, Sodium: 78mg

▶ **serving suggestions**
▪ These breadcrumbs can be used as a garnish, adding flavor and crunch to recipes such as Chicken Cordon Bleu Roll-Ups (page 33), 3-C Casserole (page 110), and Turkey Cheddar Roll-Ups (page 38).
▪ You can also use them as a substitute for regular breadcrumbs in favorite family recipes for meatloaf or meatballs.

crunchy toppings

▶ **ESTIMATED PREPARATION TIME:** 2 minutes ▶ **COOK TIME:** none ▶ **SERVINGS:** 2 cups (32 1-tablespoon servings)

These toppings can give slow cooked foods a needed crunch. They're easy to
make and handy to have on hand. The Soy Nut Topping is great on salads.

pork rind topping:
2 ounces fried pork rind snacks

or

soy nut topping:
7-ounce bag roasted, salted soy nuts

1. Add the topping of your choice to a large zip-top bag; seal the bag. Using a rolling pin, roll over the bag, crushing the soy nuts or pork rinds into small crumbs.
2. Store in the bag, or in another airtight container.

approximate nutritional content of Pork Rind Topping
▶ Calories: 10, Protein: 1g, Net Carbs: 0g, Fat: 1g, Cholesterol: 2mg, Sodium: 33mg

approximate nutritional content of Soy Nut Topping
▶ Calories: 30, Protein: 2g, Net Carbs: 1g, Fat: 2g, Cholesterol: 0mg, Sodium: 28mg

parmesan and garlic croutons

▶ **ESTIMATED PREPARATION TIME:** 5 minutes   ▶ **COOK TIME:** 50 minutes in oven   ▶ **SERVINGS:** 9 (8 croutons per serving)

These are a great addition to salads and also give soups some crunch and extra flavor. My kids like these as a snack eaten out-of-hand. If you like them that way, limit yourself or they'll be gone in no time and your carb count will be off for the day! —KB

3 tablespoons butter, melted
3 tablespoons olive oil
1 teaspoon garlic powder
½ teaspoon kosher salt
¼ teaspoon black pepper
⅓ cup grated Parmesan cheese
8 slices low-carb bread, crusts removed
   and discarded

1. Preheat oven to 300°F. In a large mixing bowl, combine all ingredients, except the bread; set aside. Cut each slice of bread into 9 rectangular pieces.

2. Add bread pieces to the mixing bowl and toss until they're well-coated with mixture. Turn the seasoned croutons out onto a baking sheet.

3. Bake at 300°F for 20 minutes, then turn oven up to 325°F and bake another 15 minutes. Using a metal spatula, flip croutons on the baking sheet and bake an additional 15 minutes.

4. Turn off the oven and let croutons cool in the oven. Store cooled croutons in an airtight container.

approximate nutritional content
   ▶ Calories: 152, Protein: 8g, Net Carbs: 3g, Fat: 11g, Cholesterol: 13mg, Sodium: 235mg

giant soup croutons

▶ **ESTIMATED PREPARATION TIME:** 5 minutes ▶ **COOK TIME:** 30 minutes in oven ▶ **SERVINGS:** 8

Perfect for French Onion Soup (page 58) or any other soup that deserves a yummy crouton!

5 tablespoons butter, melted
8 slices low-carb bread, crusts removed
½ teaspoon kosher salt
½ teaspoon black pepper

1. Preheat oven to 325°F. Using a pastry brush, brush the melted butter onto both sides of each piece of bread. Place bread slices onto a cookie sheet. Sprinkle each with salt and pepper.
2. Bake for 15 minutes, then flip bread over and continue to bake another 10 to 15 minutes, until nicely browned.
3. Let croutons cool on a cooling rack, and store in an airtight container.

approximate nutritional content
▶ Calories: 134, Protein: 7g, Net Carbs: 3g, Fat: 9g, Cholesterol: 19mg, Sodium: 223mg

▶ **serving suggestion**
For a great addition to a salad or soup, do like the restaurants do, and spread the croutons with goat cheese, then broil until the cheese is heated through.

cucumber-yogurt dressing

▶ **ESTIMATED PREPARATION TIME:** 5 minutes ▶ **COOK TIME:** none (refrigerate at least 1 hour, and overnight is preferable) ▶ **SERVINGS:** 6

This is a tangy dressing that's perfect over chopped tomatoes. For an added twist, toss in a tablespoon of chopped fresh mint leaves.

1 cup whole milk plain yogurt

1 cucumber, peeled, seeded and finely chopped

1 teaspoon fresh minced garlic

1 tablespoon extra virgin olive oil

1½ teaspoons dried minced onions

⅓ teaspoon Tabasco sauce (about 2 shakes)

1. In a medium mixing bowl, whisk together all ingredients. Cover with plastic wrap and refrigerate at least 1 hour, and preferably overnight, before serving.

approximate nutritional content
▶ Calories: 53, Protein: 2g, Net Carbs: 3.5g, Fat: 4g, Cholesterol: 5mg, Sodium: 22mg

> ▶ **about the ingredients**
> We prefer Stonyfield Farm yogurt because it's organic, and tastes great, and some varieties also contain inulin. Inulin is a natural dietary fiber that's found in a variety of fruits and vegetables. Stonyfield Farm uses it both for its probiotic effects (its ability to increase the activity of the live, beneficial bacteria cultures in yogurt, and to help prevent the growth of harmful bacteria in the human digestive tract), and because it increases our absorption of the yogurt's calcium. To low-carbers, the increased fiber provided by the inulin means fewer net carbs—always a good thing!

sesame-soy dressing for green vegetables

▶ **ESTIMATED PREPARATION TIME:** 5 minutes   ▶ **COOK TIME:** none (refrigerate overnight)   ▶ **SERVINGS:** 16

My sister-in-law Rose Regan, who loves Asian flavors, introduced me to this recipe. It has since become one of my favorite staple recipes. It's very easy to make and really jazzes up green veggies. —KM

½ cup plus 1 tablespoon soy sauce

1 tablespoon plus 1 teaspoon Splenda Granular sweetener

¼ cup rice vinegar

1 teaspoon kosher salt

¼ cup sesame oil

1. In a small mixing bowl, whisk together all ingredients. Cover with plastic wrap and refrigerate overnight.
2. Let dressing warm up to room temperature before serving (pour out the estimated amount you'll need and let that sit out; put the remainder back in the refrigerator).

approximate nutritional content
▶ Calories: 33, Protein: 0.5g, Net Carbs: 0g, Fat: 3g, Cholesterol: 0mg, Sodium: 324mg

▶ **cook's tip**
This is an intensely flavored dressing. A little goes a long way!

▶ **serving suggestion**
This dressing is wonderful served over blanched green beans, blanched asparagus, or wilted fresh spinach. It's also great over pan-fried tofu. Sprinkle toasted sesame seeds on top for interest and texture!

side dishes: salads and vegetables

marinated tomato and feta salad

▶ **ESTIMATED PREPARATION TIME:** 5 minutes ▶ **COOK TIME:** none (refrigerate at least 8 hours) ▶ **SERVINGS:** 4

An easy, make-ahead salad that pairs well with slow cooked entrées.

½ medium onion, sliced into 1-inch strips

¼ teaspoon kosher salt

¼ teaspoon black pepper

½ cup crumbled feta cheese (2 ounces)

¼ teaspoon oregano

½ cup chopped black olives

1 pint cherry tomatoes, halved (quartered, if they're very large)

½ cup bottled Greek salad dressing

1 6-ounce bag baby spinach

1. In a plastic bowl, layer onions, salt and pepper, feta, oregano, olives, and tomatoes. Pour dressing over top. Cover bowl and refrigerate at least 8 hours or overnight. Do not stir; the dressing will filter through the salad ingredients.

2. To serve, divide baby spinach among individual plates. Toss the tomato mixture thoroughly and spoon onto baby spinach.

approximate nutritional content
▶ Calories: 196, Protein: 8g, Net Carbs: 6g, Fat: 16g, Cholesterol: 36mg, Sodium: 764mg

jen's broccoli salad

▶ **ESTIMATED PREPARATION TIME:** 15 minutes ▶ **COOK TIME:** none ▶ **SERVINGS:** 6

My friend Jen Hobbs modified a family recipe to fit into her husband's low-carb diet. We think you'll agree that the result is a success! Bring it to your next picnic or BBQ party. —KM

½ cup bacon pieces (about 4 slices bacon, cooked and chopped)

½ cup sunflower seeds

½ medium red onion, finely chopped

1 cup mayonnaise

2 tablespoons cider vinegar

¼ cup Splenda Granular sweetener

½ teaspoon Worcestershire sauce

¼ teaspoon kosher salt

⅛ teaspoon black pepper

1 bunch fresh broccoli, stems chopped, crowns separated into small florets (about 4 cups)

1. In a large mixing bowl, combine all ingredients, except for broccoli; mix well. Add broccoli pieces and mix well to coat with the dressing.

2. Refrigerate salad until serving time.

approximate nutritional content
▶ Calories: 374, Protein: 6g, Net Carbs: 5g, Fat: 37g, Cholesterol: 25mg, Sodium: 318mg

EASY SUBSTITUTION

Toasted slivered almonds are a nice substitute for the sunflower seeds. This does not alter the nutritional content.

▶ **cook's tip**

This salad tastes best if refrigerated for 3 to 4 hours before serving.

---

warm asparagus and red pepper salad

▶ **ESTIMATED PREPARATION TIME:** 5 minutes   ▶ **COOK TIME:** 6 minutes   ▶ **SERVINGS:** 4

There are never any leftovers when I make this salad. Serving the vegetables warm or even at room temperature really brings out the bold flavors. —KM

2 tablespoons extra-virgin olive oil

1 large red bell pepper, cut into ¼-inch-thick slices, then cut into bite-sized pieces

1 pound fresh asparagus, trimmed and cut into 1-inch pieces

½ teaspoon kosher salt

¼ teaspoon black pepper

1 tablespoon red wine vinegar

¼ cup shredded or shaved Parmesan cheese

1. In a large skillet, over medium heat, warm olive oil; add red pepper, asparagus, salt, and pepper. Sauté until asparagus is tender but still crisp, about 5 minutes.

2. Add vinegar to skillet and stir to combine with vegetables. Remove from heat and transfer mixture to a serving dish; cool slightly.

3. Top vegetables with the Parmesan cheese and serve while still warm.

approximate nutritional content
▶ Calories: 101, Protein: 4g, Net Carbs: 4g, Fat: 8g, Cholesterol: 3mg, Sodium: 90mg

tomato, basil, and fresh mozzarella salad

▶ **ESTIMATED PREPARATION TIME:** 10 minutes   ▶ **COOK TIME:** none   ▶ **SERVINGS:** 6

Using your favorite brand of prepared pesto makes this salad super-easy to prepare, and with all the bright flavors, no one will ever guess that you didn't make it all from scratch!

⅓ cup prepared pesto

¾ pound fresh mozzarella balls, drained, sliced, and patted dry

1 pound vine-ripened tomatoes (about 4), cored and sliced thick

1 tablespoons good-quality, extra-virgin olive oil

1 teaspoon balsamic vinegar

¼ teaspoon kosher salt

¼ teaspoon black pepper

toasted pine nuts (optional)

1. Using a butter knife, spread pesto onto the cheese slices. On a platter, layer the mozzarella slices with the tomato slices. Drizzle the oil and vinegar over all.
2. Sprinkle with salt and pepper and garnish with toasted pine nuts, if desired.

approximate nutritional content
▶ Calories: 282, Protein: 15g, Net Carbs: 7g, Fat: 21g, Cholesterol: 44mg, Sodium: 415mg

faux potato salad

▶ **ESTIMATED PREPARATION TIME:** 10 minutes ▶ **COOK TIME:** none (best if refrigerated overnight) ▶ **SERVINGS:** 6

This is a great dish to bring along to a cookout or picnic; people will love it and you'll never miss the real thing.

⅔ cup mayonnaise

2 teaspoons white vinegar

2 teaspoons brown mustard

1 teaspoon celery salt

½ teaspoon black pepper

¼ teaspoon Tabasco sauce (about 2 shakes)

3 hard-boiled eggs, peeled and chopped

½ cup bacon pieces (about 6 pieces bacon, cooked and chopped)

1 1-pound bag frozen cauliflower, thawed and cut into bite-sized pieces

½ medium red onion, finely chopped

1. In a large mixing bowl, combine the first 6 ingredients (mayonnaise through Tabasco sauce); whisk well. Using a wooden spoon, gently stir in the eggs, bacon, cauliflower, and onion, so all ingredients are coated with the dressing. Refrigerate overnight for best flavor.

approximate nutritional content
▶ Calories: 260, Protein: 7g, Net Carbs: 4g, Fat: 24g, Cholesterol: 124mg, Sodium: 671mg

kim's mom's cucumber salad

▶ **ESTIMATED PREPARATION TIME:** 10 minutes ▶ **COOK TIME:** (refrigerate at least 1 hour; overnight is fine)
▶ **SERVINGS:** 4

Kim's mother, Patricia Sundik, is an avid gardener, so cukes are plentiful around
her house every summer. This cool and tangy salad is the perfect complement to a slow
cooked meal—and an easy way to make use of summer's bounty.

½ cup water

6 tablespoons white vinegar

3 teaspoons Splenda Granular sweetener

½ teaspoon kosher salt

¼ teaspoon black pepper

1 large cucumber, peeled, seeded, and cut
    into ¼-inch-thick slices

10 radishes, thinly sliced

⅓ cup grated carrot

1. In a liquid measuring cup, measure the water. Add the next 4 ingredients to the measuring cup (vinegar through pepper) and stir together to make the dressing.
2. In a medium, nonreactive (plastic or ceramic) mixing bowl, combine the vegetables. Pour dressing over all and stir to combine. Cover the salad with plastic wrap and refrigerate for at least 1 hour.
3. Prior to serving, drain excess dressing off the salad.

approximate nutritional content
▶ Calories: 19, Protein: 1g, Net Carbs: 4g, Fat: 0g, Cholesterol: 0mg, Sodium: 67mg

zippy coleslaw

▶ **ESTIMATED PREPARATION TIME:** 10 minutes ▶ **COOK TIME:** none (dressing needs to be refrigerated overnight)
▶ **SERVINGS:** 8

This recipe is a great break from creamy coleslaw and has a zippy flavor that's
bright and refreshing when paired with slow cooked foods.

½ medium onion, finely chopped

½ cup vegetable oil

⅓ cup cider vinegar

⅓ cup Splenda Granular sweetener

¾ teaspoon celery salt

⅓ cup brown mustard

¼ teaspoon Tabasco sauce (about 2
shakes)

1 1-pound bag cabbage coleslaw mix

1. In a small bowl, combine all ingredients except for the
   cabbage; cover and refrigerate overnight.
2. Just before serving, toss the dressing with the coleslaw
   mix in a large bowl and serve cold.

approximate nutritional content
   ▶ Calories: 151, Protein: 2g, Net Carbs: 4g, Fat: 15g,
   Cholesterol: 0mg, Sodium: 439mg

creamy coleslaw

▶ **ESTIMATED PREPARATION TIME:** 5 minutes ▶ **COOK TIME:** none (dressing needs be refrigerated at least 6 hours; overnight is fine) ▶ **SERVINGS:** 4

Packaged shredded cabbage and coleslaw "mix" is available at nearly every grocery store. This easy recipe complements many of our heartier meat dishes nicely, especially the BBQ Short Ribs (page 92).

⅓ cup mayonnaise

¼ cup Splenda Granular sweetener

3 tablespoons plus 1 teaspoon white vinegar

¼ teaspoon celery salt

1 shake Tabasco sauce

1 8-ounce bag shredded cabbage coleslaw mix

1. In a small bowl, combine all ingredients, except for the coleslaw mix; cover and refrigerate at least 6 hours, preferably overnight.
2. The next day, toss the dressing with the coleslaw mix in a large bowl and serve cold.

approximate nutritional content
   ▶ Calories: 133, Protein: 1g, Net Carbs: 3g, Fat: 13g, Cholesterol: 10mg, Sodium: 239mg

---

▶ **cook's tip**

This recipe doubles easily for parties and cookouts, so invite your neighbors! Also, if you prefer, you can substitute broccoli slaw for the cabbage coleslaw mix. To do so will change the approximate nutritional content to:

   ▶ Calories: 135, Protein: 2g, Net Carbs: 3g, Fat: 13g, Cholesterol: 10mg, Sodium: 244mg

asian broccoli slaw

▶ **ESTIMATED PREPARATION TIME:** 5 minutes ▶ **COOK TIME:** none (dressing needs to be refrigerated overnight)
▶ **SERVINGS:** 4

This salad will be a favorite for parties, plus it's easy to make and goes great
with many slow cooked foods. Both children and adults seem to like it as a change of
pace from the usual salad.

½ teaspoon minced ginger

¼ teaspoon garlic powder

¼ cup sesame oil

¼ cup vegetable oil

¼ cup rice wine vinegar

2 teaspoons Splenda Granular sweetener

¼ teaspoon Tabasco sauce (about 2 shakes)

1 tablespoon soy sauce

1 12-ounce package broccoli slaw

½ cup toasted sliced almonds (about 2 ounces)

1. In a small bowl, whisk together all ingredients, except for the broccoli slaw and almonds, and refrigerate overnight to combine flavors.

2. Just before serving, toss the broccoli slaw, almonds, and dressing together in a serving bowl. (You may want to use only some of the dressing, for a "drier" slaw.)

approximate nutritional content
▶ Calories: 337, Protein: 5g, Net Carbs: 3.5g, Fat: 34g, Cholesterol: 0mg, Sodium: 283mg

---

▶ **about the ingredients**

Broccoli slaw can be found in many grocery stores, right next to the packaged cabbage slaw in the produce section. It's made from shredded broccoli stems and is a healthy and unique way to serve broccoli. Try topping broccoli slaw with your favorite Italian dressing for a quick side dish on a busy night.

▶ **cook's tips**

▪ If you don't have rice wine vinegar, you can substitute white wine vinegar or regular white distilled vinegar, and the slaw will be just as tasty.

▪ You can also make this slaw with packaged coleslaw mix (cabbage) if you like.

warm spinach salad

▶ **ESTIMATED PREPARATION TIME:** 10 minutes ▶ **COOK TIME:** 5 minutes ▶ **SERVINGS:** 4

A unexpected alternative to regular spinach salad. This salad is also a tasty way to get more greens into your diet.

3 tablespoons olive oil
½ medium red onion, finely chopped
1 teaspoon kosher salt
½ teaspoon black pepper
1 teaspoon Splenda Granular sweetener
3 tablespoons cider vinegar
1 tablespoon Dijon mustard
¼ cup chopped cooked bacon
8 ounces prewashed spinach (thick stems removed), chopped into bite-sized pieces
chopped hard-boiled egg (optional)
toasted chopped almonds (optional)

1. Place spinach in a serving bowl; set aside.
2. In a medium skillet, over medium heat, warm olive oil; add onion, salt, and pepper. Cook, stirring, until onion is soft, about 3 minutes. Add all remaining ingredients, except spinach and garnishes. Stir well and cook until heated through.
3. Pour warm dressing over the spinach and toss to coat spinach with dressing. Garnish with chopped egg or toasted almonds, if desired.

approximate nutritional content
▶ Calories: 135, Protein: 3g, Net Carbs: 3g, Fat: 12g, Cholesterol: 3mg, Sodium: 311mg

super-delish snap peas

▶ **ESTIMATED PREPARATION TIME:** 8 minutes ▶ **COOK TIME:** 6 minutes ▶ **SERVINGS:** 4

The season for snap peas is so fleeting, you should take advantage of it when you find them at local farmer's markets or your supermarket. This simple recipe highlights their fresh flavor.

2 tablespoons butter, divided
1½ pounds fresh snap peas, cleaned and strings pulled
½ tablespoon kosher salt
¼ teaspoon black pepper

1. In a large skillet, over medium heat, melt 1 tablespoon of the butter; add peas, salt, and pepper. Sauté until tender but still crisp, about 5 minutes.
2. Turn off the heat; add remaining 1 tablespoon butter, toss, and serve.

approximate nutritional content
▶ Calories: 119, Protein: 5g, Net Carbs: 0g, Fat: 6g, Cholesterol: 16mg, Sodium: 245mg

summer squash sauté

▶ **ESTIMATED PREPARATION TIME:** 10 minutes   ▶ **COOK TIME:** 15 minutes   ▶ **SERVINGS:** 5

This summer side dish pairs really well with tomato-based meat dishes, as well as seafood.

2 pounds summer squash or zucchini (about 4 small)

1 tablespoon olive oil

1 tablespoon butter

½ medium onion, thinly sliced

2 teaspoons minced garlic

½ teaspoon kosher salt

½ teaspoon black pepper

¼ teaspoon Tabasco sauce (about 2 shakes)

¼ cup grated Parmesan

1. Wash and cut squash into half-moon slices about ¼-inch thick; set aside.

2. In a large skillet, warm olive oil; add butter and stir to melt. Add onions, garlic, salt, and pepper to the skillet and cook for 3 to 4 minutes, or until softened and fragrant.

3. Add the squash and Tabasco sauce to the skillet and cook, stirring, about 8 to 10 minutes, or until squash is softened. Stir in Parmesan cheese and serve hot.

approximate nutritional content
▶ Calories: 108, Protein: 4g, Net Carbs: 5g, Fat: 7g, Cholesterol: 10mg, Sodium: 170mg

sautéed baby spinach

▶ **ESTIMATED PREPARATION TIME:** 2 minutes ▶ **COOK TIME:** 5 minutes ▶ **SERVINGS:** 2

An easy, nutritious side dish. Feel free to substitute a 16-ounce bag of regular fresh spinach if baby spinach is not available; just be sure to remove any large stems and roughly chop the spinach leaves.

1 tablespoon olive oil

2 6-ounce bags baby spinach, rinsed and picked through

2 teaspoons minced garlic

¼ teaspoon kosher salt

¼ teaspoon black pepper

1. In a large skillet, over medium heat, warm the olive oil; add the garlic and heat until fragrant.
2. Add the spinach, salt, and pepper to the skillet and stir until spinach is wilted and coated with garlic, about 2 minutes. Serve hot.

approximate nutritional content
▶ Calories: 102, Protein: 5g, Net Carbs: 2g, Fat: 7g, Cholesterol: 0mg, Sodium: 195mg

green beans with bacon

▶ **ESTIMATED PREPARATION TIME:** 10 minutes　▶ **COOK TIME:** 8 minutes　▶ **SERVINGS:** 6

One taste of this dish and you'll know that green beans and bacon were destined to be together!

2 tablespoons olive oil

8 slices of cooked bacon, chopped

½ medium onion, thinly sliced

½ teaspoon kosher salt

¼ teaspoon black pepper

1½ pounds fresh green beans, trimmed and cut in half crosswise (or frozen beans, thawed)

1. In a large skillet, over medium heat, warm olive oil; add bacon, onion, salt, and pepper. Sauté until onion is softened, about 3 minutes.

2. Add beans to the pan and continue to sauté until beans are tender but still crisp, about 4 minutes.

approximate nutritional content
▶ Calories: 125, Protein: 5g, Net Carbs: 5g, Fat: 9g, Cholesterol: 7mg, Sodium: 182mg

green beans with butter and hot sauce

▶ **ESTIMATED PREPARATION TIME:** 5 minutes ▶ **COOK TIME:** 10 minutes ▶ **SERVINGS:** 6

This is one of my signature side dishes. Do not let the amount of Tabasco scare you—the beans are not overly spicy, just yummy. —KM

2 tablespoons butter, divided

1 1-pound bag frozen French-cut green beans (no need to thaw)

½ teaspoon black pepper

¼ teaspoon kosher salt

1 teaspoon Tabasco sauce (or more, if desired)

1. In a large skillet, over medium heat, add 1 tablespoon of the butter. When melted and bubbling, add the green beans, salt, and pepper; stir.
2. Continue to cook over medium heat while stirring, until green beans reach desired doneness (about 8–10 minutes).
3. When done, add remaining butter and Tabasco sauce and stir well.

approximate nutritional content
▶ Calories: 57, Protein: 1g, Net Carbs: 3g, Fat: 4g, Cholesterol: 10mg, Sodium: 67mg

▶ **cook's tip**
You may use an equal amount of fresh green beans instead of the frozen ones, but the cooking time may be a bit longer.

broccoli rabe with pine nuts

▶ **ESTIMATED PREPARATION TIME:** 5 minutes ▶ **COOK TIME:** 5 minutes ▶ **SERVINGS:** 4

Broccoli rabe is a leafy green that's very popular in Italian cuisine. If it's unavailable at your market, you can substitute fresh spinach or mustard greens.

1 bunch (about 12 ounces) broccoli rabe
  (also called rapini)
2 tablespoons extra-virgin olive oil
¼ cup pine nuts
1 tablespoon fresh minced garlic
¼ teaspoon kosher salt
½ teaspoon black pepper

1. Cut the stems away from the broccoli rabe and discard. Roughly chop the greens, and set aside.
2. In a large skillet, over medium heat, warm olive oil; add pine nuts and toast them in the oil about 1 minute, until they turn golden brown. Add garlic and sauté until fragrant.
3. Add broccoli rabe (including the greens), salt, and pepper; continue to cook until rabe is wilted (about 1–2 minutes). Toss all ingredients together before serving.

approximate nutritional content
  ▶ Calories: 120, Protein: 5g, Net Carbs: 5.5g, Fat: 10g, Cholesterol: 0mg, Sodium: 52mg

EASY ADD-INS
  ▪ Add some spice with ½ teaspoon crushed red pepper flakes.
  ▪ To make the dish more substantial, top the warm broccoli rabe with slices of fresh mozzarella cheese.

▶ **cook's tip**
Freshly minced garlic is best in this recipe, but minced garlic from a jar will also work.

desserts

peanut butter fudge cake with peanut butter drizzle

▶ **ESTIMATED PREPARATION TIME:** 10 minutes ▶ **COOK TIME:** 1½ hours (plus 1 hour cooling time) ▶ **SERVINGS:** 10

Peanut butter and chocolate have been friends forever. This special-occasion recipe brings these two favorites together again. —KM

for the cake:
2 teaspoons butter
⅓ cup smooth peanut butter
⅓ cup hot water
2 eggs, beaten
½ teaspoon vanilla
1 8.5-ounce package low-carb brownie
    mix

for the peanut butter drizzle:
½ cup half-and-half
⅓ cup smooth peanut butter
3 tablespoons Splenda Granular sweetener
½ teaspoon vanilla

1. Grease the slow cooker crock with the butter; set aside.
2. In a large mixing bowl, whisk together the peanut butter and hot water; add the eggs and vanilla and whisk well. Stir in the brownie mix using a wooden spoon. Drop the batter, by spoonfuls, into the center of the slow cooker crock (depending on the size of slow cooker you're using, it may or may not completely cover the bottom—that's okay).
3. Cover and cook on HIGH for 1 hour. Carefully remove the slow cooker lid (so as not to drip on the cake) and test for doneness using a toothpick (the pick should come out clean). If not done, wipe condensed water off inside of slow cooker lid, re-cover and cook ½ hour more on HIGH. When done, remove the slow cooker lid and lift out the crock. Allow the cake to cool in the crock, uncovered, for at least an hour before serving.
4. Just before serving, prepare the peanut butter drizzle: In a small saucepan, combine the half-and-half, peanut butter, and Splenda over low heat. Whisk and cook until peanut butter is melted and mixture is smooth. Remove from heat, whisk in the vanilla, and immediately drizzle over individual servings of cake. If drizzle gets thick, it can be reheated over low heat on the stove.

approximate nutritional content
▶ Calories: 196, Protein: 7g, Net Carbs: 19g, Fat: 11g, Cholesterol: 49mg, Sodium: 116mg

▶ **cook's tip**
A convenient way to prepare this dish for company is to put the ingredients together and start the slow cooker when guests arrive. By the time you're ready for dessert a couple of hours later, you'll need only prepare the peanut butter drizzle and serve.

coconut custard

▶ **ESTIMATED PREPARATION TIME:** 10 minutes   ▶ **COOK TIME:** 3 hours (plus 1 hour to cool in slow cooker)
▶ **SERVINGS:** 8

If you like coconut, you'll love this dessert! If you can, make it a day ahead of time—it's even better served straight from the refrigerator.

2 teaspoons butter

3 cups half-and-half

1 cup canned coconut milk

5 eggs, beaten

1 teaspoon vanilla

1 cup Splenda Granular sweetener

2 cups unsweetened, shredded coconut

pinch kosher salt

$\frac{1}{4}$ teaspoon coconut extract

whipped cream (optional)

toasted, unsweetened coconut (optional)

1. Grease the slow cooker crock with the butter (leave excess in the crock); set aside. In a medium mixing bowl, combine all ingredients except whipped cream and toasted coconut; mix well and pour into the slow cooker crock.

2. Cover and cook on LOW for 3 hours. At the end of the cooking time, give the slow cooker a gentle jiggle to make sure the custard is set (you can also gently touch the top of the custard with your finger or the back of a spoon to test it). If it's not set, cook $\frac{1}{2}$ hour more. If it is set, leave the crock uncovered and let the custard sit for 1 hour at room temperature.

3. Slice the custard and use a pie server to remove each piece (the first piece will be difficult to remove in one piece; after that it should be easy.) Garnish custard with whipped cream and a sprinkling of toasted coconut, if desired. Refrigerate any leftovers.

approximate nutritional content
▶ Calories: 266, Protein: 13g, Net Carbs: 8g, Fat: 20g, Cholesterol: 328mg, Sodium: 170mg

---

▶ **serving suggestions**

■ Top each portion with a drizzle of Low-Carb Hot Fudge (page 213) sauce.

■ For easy entertaining, make the custard a day ahead and, before refrigerating it, spoon it into individual dessert cups or ramekins. They'll be ready to garnish and serve in a snap the next day!

▶ **about the ingredients**
Unsweetened coconut, found in health food stores, is essential here because the sweetened kind is just not low-carb.

classic egg custard

▶ **ESTIMATED PREPARATION TIME:** 10 minutes ▶ **COOK TIME:** 4 hour, (plus 1 hour to cool in slow cooker)
▶ **SERVINGS:** 6

This simple dessert is extra-nice when topped with a sprinkle of nutmeg, cinnamon, or a drizzle of Spiked Strawberry Sauce (page 212) and sliced strawberries.

2 teaspoons softened butter

8 eggs, well beaten

2 cups half-and-half

2 cups whole milk

1 cup Splenda Granular sweetener

ground cinnamon or nutmeg (optional)

whipped cream (optional)

1. Grease the slow cooker crock with the butter (leave excess in the crock); set aside.
2. In a medium mixing bowl, combine all ingredients except cinnamon and whipped cream; mix well and pour into the slow cooker crock.
3. Cover and cook on LOW for 4 hours. At the end of the cooking time, give the slow cooker a gentle jiggle to make sure the custard is set (you can also gently touch the top of the custard with your finger or the back of a spoon to test it). If it's not set, cook ½ hour more. If it is set, leave the crock uncovered and let the custard sit for 1 hour at room temperature.
4. Slice the custard and use a pie server to remove each piece (the first piece will be difficult to remove in one piece; after that it should be easy). Garnish custard with a sprinkle of cinnamon or nutmeg and a dollop of whipped cream, if desired. Refrigerate any leftovers.

approximate nutritional content
▶ Calories: 266, Protein: 13g, Net Carbs: 8g, Fat: 20g, Cholesterol: 328mg, Sodium: 170mg

▶ **cook's tip**

If your custard pieces all break up as you serve them, simply switch from plates to bowls and call it "country custard"—no one will be the wiser.

pumpkin pudding with whipped cream

ESTIMATED PREPARATION TIME: 10 minutes ▸ **COOK TIME:** 3 hour, (plus cooling time) ▸ **SERVINGS:** 6

Like pumpkin pie without the crust—delish! —KB

for the pudding:

1 teaspoon butter

1 15-ounce can pumpkin (not pumpkin pie mix)

4 eggs, beaten

1½ cups half-and-half

⅔ cup Splenda Granular sweetener

1 teaspoon cinnamon

1 teaspoon vanilla

pinch salt

pinch ground cloves (optional)

pinch nutmeg (optional)

for the whipped cream:

1 cup heavy cream

2 tablespoons Splenda Granular sweetener

cinnamon (optional)

1. Grease the slow cooker crock with the butter. In a large mixing bowl, combine remaining pudding ingredients and mix well. Pour into slow cooker crock.

2. Cover and cook on LOW for 3 hours. Transfer crock to the refrigerator to cool until serving time.

3. Just before serving, prepare the whipped cream: In the bowl of an electric mixer, beat the heavy cream on medium-high speed until medium-stiff. Add Splenda and beat briefly to combine well.

4. To serve, spoon pudding into individual footed ice cream dishes or dessert bowls. Top each serving with a dollop of whipped cream and a small sprinkle of ground cinnamon, if desired.

approximate nutritional content

▸ Calories: 260, Protein: 3g, Net Carbs: 3g, Fat: 27g, Cholesterol: 146mg, Sodium: 54mg

vanilla ice cream base

▶ **ESTIMATED PREPARATION TIME:** 10 minutes ▶ **COOK TIME:** 3 hours ▶ **SERVINGS:** 16 (½-cup servings finished ice cream)

Missing ice cream? This is a simple way to make your own at home, for a lot less money than commercial low-carb ice cream, too! You will need an ice cream freezer of some kind in order to get a good-quality finished product. If you'll be living low-carb for a while (or forever), consider investing in an ice cream maker—you'll never have to miss out on this treat again!

2 cups half-and-half
1 cup Splenda Granular sweetener
pinch salt
4 egg yolks
4 cups heavy cream
1½ teaspoons pure vanilla extract (not imitation)

1. Mix all ingredients together in the slow cooker crock. Cover and cook on LOW for 2½ hours, whisking several times during cooking.
2. When cooking is complete, test to be sure it's ready using the "wooden spoon test." Dip a clean wooden spoon into the mixture, then run a clean finger over the back of the spoon (through the mixture). If your finger leaves a "trail" then the base is done. If no "trail," cook ½ hour more and test again.
3. Transfer the ice cream base to a bowl and let it cool completely in the refrigerator. Freeze ice cream according to ice cream freezer manufacturer's directions.

approximate nutritional content
▶ Calories: 260, Protein: 3g, Net Carbs: 3g, Fat: 27g, Cholesterol: 146mg, Sodium: 54mg

---

▶ **cook's tips**
▪ Because there is no added sugar in this ice cream base, it freezes very quickly and stays very hard when frozen. You may want to soften it slightly before serving.
▪ Save your egg whites for an omelet breakfast after making this recipe!
▪ This ice cream base also makes a great vanilla sauce for fresh berries.

▶ **serving suggestion**
Try topping the finished ice cream with our Low-Carb Hot Fudge (page 213) or Berry Sauce (page 211) and a dollop of whipped cream for a "safe" sundae.

berry sauce

▶ **ESTIMATED PREPARATION TIME:** 5 minutes ▶ **COOK TIME:** 3 hours ▶ **SERVINGS:** 16

Take advantage of in-season berries with this delicious recipe. Alternatively, frozen berries work just fine and you needn't thaw them first (but increase cooking time to 4 hours).

1 pound fresh blueberries, rinsed and picked over (about 3½ cups)

1 pound fresh strawberries, rinsed and roughly chopped (about 3½ cups)

2 tablespoons quick-cooking tapioca

½ cup Splenda Granular sweetener

pinch salt

1. Combine all ingredients in the slow cooker crock; mix well.
2. Cover and cook on LOW for 3 hours, stirring several times during cooking.
3. Refrigerate any unused sauce.

approximate nutritional content
▶ Calories: 28, Protein: 0g, Net Carbs: 6g, Fat: 0g, Cholesterol: 0mg, Sodium: 25mg

▶ **cook's tip**

Commercially grown blueberries are fine for nibbling or as a cereal topper. For jams, cooking, and baking we prefer wild blueberries, and it's not just because we live in Maine! We think their more pronounced flavor holds up better in cooking. Look for frozen or canned wild blueberries in your supermarket.

▶ **serving suggestions**

▪ Spread on top of low-carb toast.

▪ Serve with cottage cheese for lunch or breakfast.

▪ Use it as a sundae topping for low-carb ice cream; top with real whipped cream.

spiked strawberry sauce

▶ **ESTIMATED PREPARATION TIME:** 10 minutes ▶ **COOK TIME:** none (sauce needs to be refrigerated 12–24 hours)
▶ **SERVINGS:** 6

It's not a slow cooked recipe, but it's perfect over ice cream made with our slow cooked homemade Vanilla Ice Cream Base (page 120). This sauce combines strawberries with a hint of flavored liqueur, to create a superb dessert sauce.

12 ounces strawberries, washed and
 roughly chopped (frozen berries are
 fine; thaw slightly first)
3 tablespoons Splenda Granular sweetener
pinch salt
1 tablespoon favorite liqueur (Grand
 Marnier, Chambord, Amaretto, etc.)

1. In a medium mixing bowl, combine all ingredients. Transfer half the mixture to a blender; puree until smooth. Pour pureed mixture back into mixing bowl and stir to combine.

2. Cover and refrigerate at least 12 hours (overnight is fine) to let flavors blend.

approximate nutritional content
 ▶ Calories: 21, Protein: 0g, Net Carbs: 3g, Fat: 0g, Cholesterol: 0mg, Sodium: 65mg

▶ **cook's tip**
Triple Sec is an economical substitute for Grand Marnier and will work fine in this recipe.

▶ **serving suggestions**
■ Drizzle over fresh mango and top with a sprinkle of chopped almonds
■ Try it over Splenda-sweetened ricotta cheese for an "adult" dessert.
■ Serve atop a low-carb brownie and top with whipped cream.

low-carb hot fudge

▶ **ESTIMATED PREPARATION TIME:** 5 minutes ▶ **COOK TIME:** 5 minutes ▶ **SERVINGS:** 8 servings

This isn't a slow cooker recipe, but it's handy to serve with some of our desserts. If you're craving chocolate, this is your answer.

4 tablespoons butter

3 squares bittersweet chocolate (not unsweetened)

½ cup Splenda Granular sweetener

½ cup half-and-half, at room temperature

¾ teaspoon vanilla

pinch salt

1. In a small saucepan, over low heat, melt butter; add chocolate and stir until melted and combined with the butter. Remove from heat.

2. Using a whisk, mix in the remaining ingredients. Serve immediately; refrigerate any unused sauce. The sauce will harden as it cools; a few seconds in the microwave will get it back to sauce consistency.

approximate nutritional content
▶ Calories: 122, Protein: 1g, Net Carbs: 5g, Fat: 12g, Cholesterol: 21mg, Sodium: 113mg

EASY ADD-IN
For a minty sauce, add ¼ teaspoon spearmint extract.

▶ **about the ingredients**
We use bittersweet chocolate here because the sauce needs some real sugar for the best flavor.

acknowledgments

MANY OF MY friends liken writing a book to giving birth, a very apt comparison in many ways. The development of this book was, like most pregnancies, filled with wonderful experiences, discoveries, and pleasures. And, for the most part, it was painless—and in that respect, very *unlike* pregnancy—or at least the delivery aspect. The ease of this "birth" is due in large part to the contributions and assistance provided to me and Kim by the following people:

- Jacqueline Marcus, who recommended me for this project. Thanks for always being a mentor, for your confidence in me, and for sharing both professionally and personally.
- Amy Barr, for introducing me to Kim at IACP. You're a great example of professional networking at its finest, and I thank you for keeping me in your Rolodex.
- Lisa Ekus, for taking a chance on the Kitty–Kim team, and for all things agent-related. We're looking forward to more projects with you on our side.
- Sue McCloskey, our editor at Marlowe & Company, for the vision to create this book, and for your encouragement, professionalism, and faith in our abilities.
- My children, Jack and Amelia Scofield, for tolerating the lack of Mommy play-time that occurs when I'm knee-deep in writing and facing deadlines.
- And last but certainly not least, my husband, Dan Scofield, for all the little things you did to help nurture me and our family as I created this book. I noticed (even if it seemed like I didn't), and am so thankful.

—KITTY BROIHIER

THIS IS MY first book, and I am brimming with excitement and gratitude, as so many people have enriched my life and this experience. I especially want to thank the following people:

- First, the incredible man whom I married, Mark Mayone. You fill my life with joy and believe in me more than I believe in myself. Thanks also for washing all the dishes (by hand!) and for evaluating all of the food (sometimes with a strained smile). You are simply the best!
- My little sous chefs, Sophia and Harrison Mayone, who waited patiently while Mommy "filled the slow cookers" day after day, all summer long. My wonderful parents, Harry and Patricia Sundik; your love and guidance are always appreciated.
- Lise Stern, my dear friend and food writing mentor. Thank you for showing me that one can be a wonderful mother and a professional at the same time. Thank you, Pam Fischer, for hiring me at Fresh Samantha, and for showing me that work should be fun. Thanks also to Barr Hogan, my creative partner in the land of juice; our marvelous food adventures still inspire me.
- Lisa Cohen, it seems like we have been friends forever. Thank you for treating me to divine dinners at all of the "hot" new restaurants that are beyond my budget; your generosity is unsurpassed. Thanks also to Karen Lucas for being my biggest cheerleader and for being the unstoppable dynamo that you are!
- Thanks to all my friends and culinary associates who contributed recipe ideas and inspiration to this book, as well as taste-tested the results for me.
- Professional thanks to Amy Barr for introducing me to Kitty, to Lisa Ekus, our agent extraordinaire, and to our fabulous editor, Sue McCloskey at Marlowe & Company.
- Finally, thank you to the grande dame of the culinary world, Julia Child. You are my idol.

—KIM MAYONE

index

adapting traditional recipes, 8
adobo seasoning, 55
almonds
    butter roasted, 136
    chicken with olives and, 105
    in curried mixed nuts, 139
    diablo, 137
    pork cutlets with Brussels sprouts, bacon, and, 120
appetizers, 153
    babaghanoush, 143
    bacon-horseradish dip, creamy, 145
    cheese and spinach dip, easy, 147
    cheese dip, easy, 146
    chicken satay bites, 151
    cocktail party meatballs, 150
    cocktail sausages, sweet and sour, 153
    cocktail sausages with bbq sauce, 154
    con queso dip, 144
    crab dip, super, 149
    kielbasa slices, sweet and sour, 155
    meatballs stroganoff, 152
    onion and spinach dip, 148
artichoke hearts
    chicken with sun-dried tomatoes and, 96
    pork with prosciutto and, 124
Asian-inspired beef ribs, 91
asparagus and red pepper salad, warm, 190

babaghanoush, 143
bacon
    in beef bourguignonne, 89
    beef stew with beans and, 61
    blt sandwich, 173
    in broccoli salad, 189
    and cheese crustless quiche, 25

    cheese dip, 146
    green beans with, 201
    -horseradish dip, creamy, 145
    in meatloaf, classic, 75
    pork cutlets with Brussels sprouts, almonds, and, 120
barley, beef stew with, 63
barley, chicken soup with, 53
bbq
    beef short ribs with green chilies, 92
    cocktail sausages, 154
    pork ribs, classic country-style, 126
beans
    beef stew with bacon and, 61
    chicken soup with tomatoes and, 54
    in chili, 67, 68, 71
    in dude ranch soup, 55
    ham soup with spinach and, 169
    in Mexican chicken, 99
    sausage soup with, 57
    vegetable soup with, 59
bean sprouts, pan-fried, 112
beef. *See also* stews
    Asian-inspired ribs, 91
    bbq short ribs with green chilies, 92
    bourguignonne, 89
    brisket, classic, 90
    corned beef and cabbage, 158
    corned beef and onion hash, 159
    in dude ranch soup, 55
    ginger garlic, over braised Napa cabbage, 88
    herbed top round roast, 83
    Mexican pot roast, 84
    pesto, with grape tomatoes and fresh mozzarella, 40
    pot roast, classic, 82

"steak bomb" casserole, 87
teriyaki, with peppers and onions, 42
in Texas chili, 70
Thai green curry, 85
with zucchini, mushrooms, and grape tomatoes, 86
beef, ground
in cheeseburger soup, 39
in cheesy mac, 81
in chili, 67
in chop suey, American, 78
in crepesagna, 156
meatballs, frozen prepared, 150, 152
meatballs and sauce, 176
in meatloaf, 74–77
shepherd's pie, 171
in stuffed bell peppers, 79
in stuffed cabbage soup, 56
and veggie pie, 80
bell peppers. *See also* roasted red peppers
and asparagus salad, warm, 190
beef stew with onions and, 62
in chicken cacciatore, 106
Italian sausage and, 46
in kielbasa slices, sweet and sour, 155
meatballs, cocktail party, 150
in Mexican chicken, 99
quiche with mushrooms and, 26
in "steak bomb" casserole, 87
stuffed, 79
teriyaki steak with onions and, 42
berry sauce, 211
blt sandwich, 173
blueberry French toast casserole, 28
bok choy, sesame tuna with shitake mushrooms and, 131
bread, low-carb, 12–14, 29
in all-beef meatloaf, 74
blt sandwich, 173
in blueberry French toast casserole, 28
buttered parmesan breadcrumbs, 180
as croutons, 182, 183
in ham and cheese strata, 23
in smoked salmon breakfast bake, 29
breakfast. *See* brunch dishes
broccoli
Asian slaw, 196
quiche, 25
rabe with pine nuts, 203
salad, Jen's, 189
broth, cooking with, 17

brunch dishes
blueberry French toast casserole, 28
egg casserole with sweet onion and sausage, 22
ham and cheese strata, 23
huevos rancheros, 24
quiches, 25–27
smoked salmon breakfast bake, 29
Brussels sprouts, pork cutlets with almonds, bacon, and, 120
butter, cooking with, 17
buttered parmesan breadcrumbs, 180
butter roasted almonds, 136

cabbage
in coleslaw, 194, 195
corned beef and, 158
ginger garlic beef over braised Napa, 88
kielbasa, onions, and, 47
smoked picnic ham with, 168
stuffed cabbage soup, 56
carbohydrates, about, xv, 12–16
cashew nuts, in curried mixed nuts, 139
cauliflower
in beef and sausage stew, 65
in cheesy mock mashed potatoes, 170
in chicken with sun-dried tomatoes and artichokes, 96
in potato salad, faux, 192
in Thai green curry beef, 85
in Thai red curry chicken, 101
3-c casserole, 110
cheddar cheese
in beef and veggie pie, 80
in cheesy mock mashed potatoes, 170
in dude ranch soup, 55
in egg casserole with sweet onion and sausage, 22
quiche, bacon and, 25
3-c casserole, 110
turkey roll-ups with cream sauce, 38
cheese. *See also* cheddar, feta, Monterey Jack, mozzarella, provolone, and ricotta cheeses
buttered parmesan breadcrumbs, 180
con queso dip, 144
dip, easy, 146
in huevos rancheros, 24
mascarpone, in chicken with exotic mushrooms, 32
parmesan and garlic croutons, 182
sauce, creamy, 177
and spinach dip, easy, 147

Swiss, in chicken cordon bleu roll-ups, 33
cheeseburger soup, 39
cheesy mac, 81
chicken
    -barley soup, 53
    cacciatore, 106
    casserole, creamy layered, 107
    and cheese strata, 23
    with Chinese black bean sauce, 112
    cordon bleu roll-ups, 33
    with exotic mushrooms, 32
    with 40 cloves of garlic, 160
    Greek, 97
    herb roasted, 35
    Italian, 95
    lemon roasted, with optional herbs, 34
    lentil, and spinach stew, Middle Eastern, 66
    margarita, 113
    marsala, 108
    martini, 102
    Mexican, 99
    with mushrooms and leeks, 94
    with olives and almonds, 105
    orange, 121
    pesto, with grape tomatoes and fresh
        mozzarella, 40
    piccata, 109
    with prosciutto and artichoke hearts, 124
    pseudo-saltimbocca, 111
    with quinoa, 103
    salad, classic, 161
    salad, Dijon ranch, 163
    salad, toasted-walnut and apple, 162
    satay bites, 151
    scallion and peanut, 100
    sofrito, 37
    soup, 52
    souvlaki, 43
    with summer vegetables, 104
    with sun-dried tomatoes and artichokes, 96
    teriyaki roasted, 36
    Thai red curry, 101
    thighs, rosemary and garlic, 98
    3-c casserole, 110
    tomato, and white bean soup, 54
    in white chili, 71
chickpeas
    beef stew with spinach and, 64
    in ciao bella chili, 69
    sausage with tomatoes and, 45
chilies. *See* green chilies

chili recipes, 67–71
chili-rubbed shredded pork, 128
chocolate
    fudge, low-carb hot, 213
    in peanut butter fudge cake with peanut butter
        drizzle, 206
chop suey, American, 78
ciao bella chili, 69
cinnamon walnuts, 138
citrus salmon, 132
cocktail sausages
    153,154
coconut custard, 207
coleslaw, creamy, 195
coleslaw, zippy, 194
con queso dip, 144
cooking spray, 7
corned beef and cabbage, 158
corned beef and onion hash, 159
country-style bbq pork ribs, classic, 126
crab dip, super, 149
cranberry and horseradish sauce with ham, 41
cream. *See also* half-and-half
    in blueberry French toast casserole, 28
    in egg casserole with sweet onion and sausage,
        22
    pumpkin pudding with whipped cream, 209
    in quiche, 25–27
    in smoked salmon breakfast bake, 29
    as topping for fruit, 111
    in vanilla ice cream base, 210
créme fraîche, in chicken with mushrooms and
    leeks, 94
crepesagna, 156
crunchy toppings, 181
cucumber salad, kim's mom's, 193
cucumber-yogurt dressing, 184
curry
    in chicken satay bites, 151
    curried mixed nuts, 139
    Thai green curry beef, 85
    Thai red curry chicken, 101

dairy products, 8. *See also* cheese; cream; half-and-
    half; sour cream
    cucumber-yogurt dressing, 184
desserts. *See also* chocolate
    berry sauce, 211
    coconut custard, 207
    egg custard, classic, 208
    pumpkin pudding with whipped cream, 209

strawberry sauce, spiked, 212
    vanilla ice cream base, 210
Dijon ranch chicken salad, 163
dressings
    cucumber-yogurt, 184
    sesame-soy, for green vegetables, 185
dude ranch soup, 55

eggplant
    babaghanoush, 143
    in vegetable sauce, 179
egg(s)
    in blueberry French toast casserole, 28
    casserole with sweet onion and sausage, 22
    custard, classic, 208
    in ham and cheese strata, 23
    hard-boiled, overnight, 164
    huevos rancheros, 24
    Italiana, 30
    pickled, 166, 167
    quiches, 25–27
    salad, classic, 165
    in smoked salmon breakfast bake, 29

fat content of recipes, 16
fennel, mixed sausage with, 44
feta cheese
    in Greek chicken, 97
    in Greek meatloaf, 76
    marinated tomato salad and, 188
fish. *See also* salmon; swordfish
    Mediterranean hake, 49
    sesame tuna (or salmon) with bok choy and
        shitake mushrooms, 131
French onion soup, 58
fruit(s)
    berry sauce, 211
    blueberry French toast casserole, 28
    strawberry sauce, spiked, 212
fudge, low-carb hot, 213

garlic, 17
    beef over braised Napa cabbage, ginger, 88
    chicken thighs, rosemary and, 98
    chicken with 40 cloves of, 160
ginger garlic beef over Napa cabbage, 88
"gravy," turkey au jus, 178
Greek chicken, 97
Greek meatloaf, 76
green beans
    with bacon, 201

    with butter and hot sauce, 202
    sesame-soy dressing for, 185
    in Thai green curry beef, 85
    in Thai red curry chicken, 101
    vegetable sauce, 179
green chilies
    bbq beef short ribs with, 92
    chili-rubbed shredded pork, 128
    in con queso dip, 144
    in dude ranch soup, 55
    in huevos rancheros, 24
    in Mexican chicken, 99
    pork chops with pecans and, 125
    in white chili, 71
green onions. *See* scallions
grocery list, 10–14, 127, 142, 151, 160, 196. *See
    also* ingredient choices

half-and-half. *See also* cream
    in cheese dip, 146, 147
    in coconut custard, 207
    in egg custard, classic, 208
    in eggs Italiana, 30
    in ham and cheese strata, 23
    in pumpkin pudding with whipped cream, 209
    in vanilla ice cream base, 210
ham. *See also* prosciutto
    and cheese strata, 23
    in chicken cordon bleu roll-ups, 33
    with cranberry and horseradish sauce, 41
    smoked picnic, with cabbage, 168
    spinach, and white bean soup, 169
hard-boiled eggs, overnight, 164
herbs
    chicken roasted with, 35
    herbed top round roast, 83
    lemon roasted chicken with, 34
    pork with roasted red peppers, olives, and, 118
    rosemary and garlic chicken thighs, 98
    tomatoes, basil, and fresh mozzarella salad, 191
high vs. low setting, 7
huevos rancheros, 24

ice cream base, vanilla, 210
ingredient choices, 17–19, 37, 85. *See also* grocery
    list
Italian chicken, 95
Italian sausage and peppers, 46

kielbasa, cabbage and onions, 47
kielbasa slices, sweet and sour, 155

kitchen tools and gadgets, 19, 35

layering foods, 8
leeks, chicken with mushrooms and, 94
leftovers, using up, 17
lemon(s), 143
    in chicken piccata, 109
    in roasted chicken, 34
    in souvlaki pork (or chicken) cutlets, 43
lentil, chicken, and spinach stew, Middle Eastern, 66
low-carb foods, sources for, 12–14
low vs. high setting, 7

macaroni, low-carb, 12–14
    American chop suey, 78
    cheesy mac, 81
maple pecans, 140
margarita chicken, 113
martini chicken, 102
measurement equivalents, 9
meatballs, frozen prepared
    cocktail party, 150
    stroganoff, 152
meatballs and sauce, 176
meats. See also bacon; beef; chicken; ham; pork
    browning, xiv, 81, 89
    purchasing, 11, 17–18
    searing, 46, 60
Mediterranean hake, 49
Mexican chicken, 99
Mexican pot roast, 84
Middle Eastern chicken, lentil, and spinach stew, 66
miso-rubbed salmon, 133
miso soup with tofu and scallions, 142
mixed sausage with fennel, 44
molasses and rum baby back ribs, 127
Monterey Jack cheese
    ham and, strata, 23
    in seafood crustless quiche, 27
    in stuffed bell peppers, 79
mozzarella cheese
    in chicken casserole, creamy layered, 107
    in crepesagna, 156
    pesto beef with grape tomatoes and fresh, 40
    tomato and basil salad with fresh, 191
mushroom(s)
    beef and barley stew, 63
    in beef and sausage stew, 65
    in beef bourguignonne, 89
    in chicken marsala, 108
    chicken with exotic, 32

chicken with leeks and, 94
    pork with scallions and shitake, 122
    quiche, red pepper and, 26
    sesame tuna with bok choy and shitake, 131
    steak with zucchini, grape tomatoes and, 86

net carbs, 16
noodles, low-carb, in chicken soup, 52
nutritional content of recipes, 15–16
nuts. See also almonds; pecans
    broccoli rabe with pine nuts, 203
    cinnamon walnuts, 138
    curried mixed nuts, 139
    scallion and peanut chicken, 100
    toasted-walnut and apple chicken salad, 162

olive oil, cooking with, 18, 132
olives, chicken with almonds and, 105
olives, pork with roasted red peppers, herbs, and, 118
onion(s), 18, 22
    beef stew with peppers and, 62
    corned beef and onion hash, 159
    egg casserole with sweet onion and sausage, 22
    French onion soup, 58
    pork smothered in, 116
    and spinach dip, 148
orange pork (or chicken), 121
oyster sauce, 100

parmesan and garlic croutons, 182
peanut butter fudge cake with peanut butter
        drizzle, 206
peanut chicken, scallion and, 100
pecans
    in curried mixed nuts, 139
    glazed sweet and spicy, 141
    maple, 140
    pork chops with chilies and, 125
peppers. See bell peppers; roasted red peppers
pesto beef with grape tomatoes and fresh
        mozzarella, 40
pickled eggs, 166, 167
pork. See also bacon; ham; prosciutto
    bbq ribs, classic country-style, 126
    chili-rubbed shredded, 128
    chops with pecans and chilies, 125
    in crepesagna, 156
    cutlets with apples and mustard, 119
    cutlets with Brussels sprouts, almonds, and
        bacon, 120
    in meatballs and sauce, 176

in meatloaf, classic, 75
orange, 121
with prosciutto and artichoke hearts, 124
with roasted red peppers, 117, 118
rum and molasses baby back ribs, 127
with scallions and shitake mushrooms, 122
smoked chops in sauerkraut, 123
smothered in onions, 116
souvlaki cutlets, 43
pork rind topping, 181
portion control, 16
potato salad, faux, 192
pot roast, 82, 84
poultry. *See* chicken; turkey
prosciutto
in chicken pseudo-saltimbocca, 111
in eggs Italiana, 30
pork with artichoke hearts and, 124
provolone cheese
in chicken pseudo-saltimbocca, 111
in eggs Italiana, 30
in "steak bomb" casserole, 87
pumpkin pudding with whipped cream, 209

quiches, 25–27
quinoa, chicken with, 103

recaito, 113
red pepper and mushroom quiche, 26
ricotta cheese
in chicken casserole, layered, 107
in crepesagna, 156
Rival Crock-Pot, xiii
roasted chicken, 35
roasted red peppers
pork with herbs, olives and, 118
pork with onions and, 117
rum and molasses baby back ribs, 127

safety with slow cookers, 5–6, 19
salads
Asian broccoli slaw, 196
asparagus and red pepper, warm, 190
broccoli, Jen's, 189
chicken, 161, 162, 163
coleslaw, 194, 195
cucumber, 193
egg, 165
marinated tomato and feta, 188
potato, faux, 192
spinach, warm, 197

tomatoes, basil, and fresh mozzarella, 191
salmon
citrus, 132
miso-rubbed, 133
sesame, with bok choy and shitake mushrooms, 131
smoked, breakfast bake, 29
salt, 18, 26, 166
sauce(s)
bbq, 154
berry, 211
cheese, creamy, 177
Chinese black bean, 112
cranberry and horseradish, 41
cream, 38
fudge, low-carb hot, 213
meatballs and, 176
strawberry, spiked, 212
vegetable (made from), 179
sauerkraut, smoked pork chops in, 123
sausage(s), 46
and beef stew, 65
with chickpeas and tomatoes, 45
in ciao bella chili, 69
cocktail, sweet and sour, 153
cocktail, with low-carb bbq sauce, 154
egg casserole with sweet onion and, 22
Italian, with peppers, 46
kielbasa, cabbage and onions, 47
kielbasa slices, sweet and sour, 155
mixed, with fennel, 44
and white bean soup, 57
scallions
miso soup with tofu and, 142
and peanut chicken, 100
pork with shitake mushrooms and, 122
seafood
cheese strata with, 23
crab dip, super, 149
quiche, crustless, 27
smoked oyster quiche, 25
sesame-soy dressing for vegetables, 185
sesame tuna with bok choy and shitake mushrooms, 131
shepherd's pie, 171
shrimp, in seafood quiche, 27
shrimp and cheese strata, 23
side dishes. *See also* salads
broccoli rabe with pine nuts, 203
cheesy mock mashed potatoes, 170
green beans with bacon, 201

green beans with butter and hot sauce, 202

snap peas, super-delish, 198

spaghetti squash, 176

spinach, sautéed baby, 200

summer squash sauté, 199

slow cookers

adapting recipes for, 8

care and safety, 4–6

types and features, 1–3

slow cooking, overview, xiii–xv, 7

smoked oyster quiche, 25

smoked picnic ham with cabbage, 168

smoked pork chops in sauerkraut, 123

smoked salmon breakfast bake, 29

smoked turkey and cheese strata, 23

snacks

almonds diablo, 137

butter roasted almonds, 136

cinnamon walnuts, 138

curried mixed nuts, 139

maple pecans, 140

pecans, glazed sweet and spicy, 141

snap peas, super-delish, 198

sofrito chicken, 37

soups. See also stews

cheeseburger, 39

chicken, tomato, and white bean, 54

chicken-barley, 53

chicken (or turkey), 52

chili recipes, 67–71

dude ranch, 55

French onion, 58, 183

ham, spinach, and white bean soup, 169

miso with tofu and scallions, 142

sausage and white bean, 57

soup croutons, giant, 183

stuffed cabbage, 56

vegetable and bean, 59

sour cream

cheesy mock mashed potatoes with, 170

in meatballs stroganoff, 152

souvlaki pork (or chicken) cutlets, 43

soy nut topping, 181

spaghetti squash, 176

spinach

beef stew with chickpeas and, 64

dip, cheese and, 147

dip, onion and, 148

in Greek meatloaf, 76

ham and white bean soup with, 169

in marinated tomato and feta salad, 188

Middle Eastern chicken, lentil, and spinach stew, 66

quiche, 25

salad, warm, 197

sautéed baby, 200

sesame-soy dressing for, 185

Splenda Granular sweetener, 18

"steak bomb" casserole, 87

steak with zucchini, mushrooms, and grape tomatoes, 86

stews. See also soups

beef, bean and bacon, 61

beef, with chickpeas and spinach, 64

beef and barley, 63

beef and sausage, 65

beef and vegetable, 60

Middle Eastern chicken, lentil, and spinach, 66

pepper and onion beef, 62

strawberry sauce, spiked, 212

summer squash, chicken with, 104

summer squash sauté, 199

sun-dried tomatoes

chicken pseudo-saltimbocca, 111

chicken with artichokes and, 96

in Greek chicken, 97

swordfish

with pesto, 130

tapenade, with tomato sauce, 48

tapenade swordfish with tomato sauce, 48

teriyaki roasted chicken, 36

teriyaki steak with peppers and onions, 42

Texas chili, 70

Thai green curry beef, 85

Thai red curry chicken, 101

3-c casserole (chicken, cheese, and cauliflower), 110

toasted-walnut and apple chicken salad, 162

tofu, miso soup with scallions and, 142

tomatoes, fresh. See also sun-dried tomatoes

basil, and fresh mozzarella salad, 191

in Greek chicken, 97

marinated, and feta salad, 188

pesto beef with grape tomatoes and fresh mozzarella, 40

steak with zucchini, mushrooms, and grape tomatoes, 86

tuna, sesame, with bok choy and shitake mushrooms, 131

turkey

blt sandwich, 173

breast, 172, 178
and cheddar roll-ups, 38
in chili, 67
smoked, and cheese strata, 23
soup, 52
in white chili, 71

vanilla ice cream base, 210
vegetable oil, cooking with, 19, 132
vegetable(s), 11, 19, 26, 60. *See also* side dishes;
    specific vegetables
asparagus and red pepper salad, warm, 190
babaghanoush (eggplant), 143
and bean soup, 59
beef and veggie pie, 80
beef stew and, 60
chicken with mushrooms and leeks, 94
chicken with summer, 104
chili, vegetarian, 68

pork cutlets with Brussels sprouts, almonds, and
    bacon, 120
sauce made from, 179
sesame-soy dressing for green, 185
sesame tuna with bok choy and shitake mush-
    rooms, 131
steak with, 86
Vidalia onions, 22

walnuts, cinnamon, 138
walnuts, toasted, and apple chicken salad, 162
warnings, safety, 5–6, 19
white chili, 71

yogurt, 184

zucchini, steak with mushrooms, grape tomatoes
    and, 86